Suicide Risk Management

A Manual for Health Professionals

DEDICATION
To our students.

Publication of this book was supported by an educational grant from Lundbeck

The Lundbeck Institute
Grevinde Danners Palae
Skodsborg Strandvej 113
DK-2942 Skodsborg
Denmark
Tel: +45 4556 0140
Fax: +45 4556 0145
E-mail: institute@lundbeck.com
Website: www.cnsforum.com

Lundbeck Institute

Suicide Risk Management

A Manual for Health Professionals

Dr Stan Kutcher
MD FRCPC
Professor of Psychiatry and Associate Dean of International Medical Development
and Research
Dalhousie University
Halifax, Canada

Dr Sonia Chehil
MD FRCPC
Assistant Professor of Psychiatry and Deputy Head of International Psychiatry
Dalhousie University
Halifax, Canada

Blackwell
Publishing

© 2007 S. Kutcher and Sonia Chehil
Published by Blackwell Publishing Ltd
Blackwell Publishing, Inc., 350 Main Street, Malden, Massachusetts 02148-5020, U
Blackwell Publishing Ltd, 9600 Garsington Road, Oxford OX4 2DQ, UK
Blackwell Publishing Asia Pty Ltd, 550 Swanston Street, Carlton, Victoria 3053, Au

The right of the Author to be identified as the Author of this Work has been asserted
accordance with the Copyright, Designs and Patents Act 1988.

First published 2007

1   2007

Library of Congress Cataloging-in-Publication Data
Kutcher, Stanley P.
  Suicide risk management : a manual for health professionals / Stan Kutcher, Sonia Chehil.
    p. ; cm.
  Includes bibliographical references and index.
  ISBN-13: 978-1-4051-5369-0
  ISBN-10: 1-4051-5369-5
  1. Suicide--Prevention. 2. Suicide--Risk factors. 3. Risk assessment.
  I. Chehil, Sonia. II. Title.
  [DNLM: 1. Suicide--prevention & control. 2. Suicide--psychology.
  3. Risk Assessment--methods.   WM 165 K97s 2006]
  RC569.K88 2006
  616.85'8445--dc22

                                                                        2006015842

ISBN-13: 978-1-4051-5369-0
ISBN-10: 1-4051-5369-5

A catalogue record for this title is available from the British Library

Set in 9/11.5 Times New Roman by Sparks, Oxford – www.sparks.co.uk
Printed and bound in Spain by GraphyCems

Commissioning Editor: Stuart Taylor
Editorial Assistant: Jenny Seward
Development Editor: Charlie Hamlyn
Production Controller: Kate Charman

For further information on Blackwell Publishing, visit our website:
http://www.blackwellpublishing.com

Contents

Introduction, vi
Objectives, viii

1 Understanding Suicide Risk, 1
2 Suicide Risk Assessment, 34
3 Putting It All Together: The Tool for Assessment of Suicide Risk (TASR), 66
4 Suicide and Youth, 71
5 Commonly Encountered Problems in the Evaluation of Suicide Risk, 80
6 Suicide Prevention, 86
7 Suicide Intervention, 88
8 Post-suicide Interventions, 93
9 Clinical Vignettes for Group or Individual Study, 96

Appendices, 113
Appendix 1 Suicide Risk Assessment Guide (SRAG), 114
Appendix 2 Tool for Assessment of Suicide Risk (TASR), 118
Appendix 3 6-item Kutcher Adolescent Depression Scale (KADS), 119
Appendix 4 Chehil and Kutcher Clinical Assessment of Adolescent Depression (CAAD), 124

Index, 131

Introduction

Understanding suicide is unachievable. The underpinnings of suicide are diverse and multifaceted, involving a unique fusion of biological, psychosocial and cultural factors for each individual. Suicide is not an event that occurs in a vacuum. It is the ultimate consequence of a process.

For many people who take the decision to end their own life we will never be able to answer the question 'Why?' For some, self-inflicted death may be:

- ...an escape from despair and suffering
- ...a relief from intractable emotional, psychological or physical pain
- ...a response to a stigmatizing illness
- ...an escape from feelings of hopelessness
- ...a consequence of acute intoxication
- ...a response to commanding homicidal or self-harm auditory hallucinations
- ...a manifestation of bizarre or grandiose delusions
- ...a declaration of religious devotion
- ...a testimony of nationalist or political allegiance
- ...a means of atonement
- ...a means of reunification with a deceased loved one
- ...a means of rebirth
- ...a method of revenge
- ...a way to protect family honour

This does not mean that health professionals should not know how to recognize, assess and manage the suicidal patient. Indeed, all health professionals should be proficient in this core competency as many of their patients may face the prospect of suicide at some time in their lives. Many patients who experience suicidal thoughts or make suicide plans will change their minds about committing suicide. Many people who attempt suicide and are not successful go on to live productive lives. For some, a suicide attempt is an event that leads to a first contact with a helping professional. Some of these individuals may be suffering from a mental disorder that will respond to appropriate and effective treatment. Some may be suffering from chronic physical disorders; others may be overwhelmed by life stressors. In any case, many of these individuals may consider suicide as a viable solution to their problems or the only means to ending their suffering. By being aware of suicide risk factors and knowing how to identify and provide appropriate targeted interventions for suicidal individuals, health professionals can assist in the patient choosing life rather than death.

Cultural, religious, geographical and socioeconomic factors all impact on the expression of suicidality and the completion of suicide. Thus, health professionals from various countries or regions may need to adapt some of the material in this book to reflect local perspectives. However, we all need to remember, whenever a clinician and a suicidal person interact, that careful, considerate application of suicide risk management will need to be applied – regardless of context. Contexts differ but people are similar.

Objectives

1 To provide information regarding the epidemiology, risk factors and associated aspects of suicide.
2 To provide information that will assist in the understanding and assessment of suicide risk.
3 To provide a continuous self-study programme pertaining to clinical evaluation of suicide, using the Suicide Risk Assessment Guide (SRAG).
4 To introduce the Tool for Assessment of Suicide Risk (TASR) and provide instruction on its appropriate clinical application.

Chapter 1
Understanding Suicide Risk

Why is it important to know about suicide?

Suicide is a significant public health problem worldwide. Estimating prevalence in different countries is problematic because in many countries suicide is hidden and therefore 'prevalence estimates' taken from national records will probably underestimate real suicide rates. In addition, different countries report marked differences in suicide rates and it is not clear why such differences occur. Nevertheless, based on available data, globally suicide is believed to account for an average of 10–15 deaths for every 100 000 persons each year, and for each completed suicide there are up to 20 failed suicide attempts. Age-adjusted suicide rates globally range from lows of 1.1/100 000 to 51.6/100 000 (WHO, 2002) but the variability of data collection makes national comparisons difficult if not impossible. In general, suicide rates in most countries have remained quite stable with the exception of Mexico, India and Brazil, where overall suicide rates have been increasing (WHO, 2001). The reasons for this are as yet poorly understood. Mortality from suicide constitutes a significant public health problem. Data from the USA indicate that reported suicide deaths are almost 40% higher than homicide deaths. Yet, much more public attention in that country focuses on homicide than on suicide.

Past data had indicated that suicide in young adults and teens had been increasing in some countries, for example in Canada and the USA. In the last decade, however, this longstanding trend has shifted. More recent data suggest that over the past decade youth suicide in some countries has actually been decreasing. In other countries rates have remained stable or may have increased somewhat. It is not clear what factors have been most important in changing these suicide rates in young people, although considerations as varied as more effective identification and treatment of depression and control of lethal means have been put forward. Nonetheless, in the USA and many other countries (particularly in wealthy or developed states), suicide continues to be one of the three leading causes of death in young people between the ages of 15 and 24.

In North America, studies indicate that the majority (up to two-thirds) of those who commit suicide have had contact with a health-care professional for various physical and emotional complaints in the month before their death. Unfortunately, many suicidal individuals may not spontaneously voice suicidal thoughts or plans of self-harm to their health-care provider, and the majority of those at risk may never be asked about suicidality during clinical assessments. It is not clear if this failure to identify suicidal individuals stems from a lack of training in the identification of those at possible risk for suicide, lack of comfort or confidence on the part of the health-care professional in addressing suicidality, time or resource constraints, or some other factors.

Psychiatric disorder is the strongest attributable risk factor for suicide.

For mental-health-care providers (such as primary care physicians, community nurses, social workers, psychologists, mental health nurses, psychiatrists and others), suicide is of particular relevance. According to some researchers, up to 90% of patients who commit suicide in Western countries may suffer from at least one major psychiatric disorder. Although there is likely to be variation in this figure across countries and cultures, it highlights the significance of the correlation between mental disorders and suicide.

What are some of the barriers to detection and prevention of suicide?

Several factors can impede the detection and prevention of suicide:
* stigma and secrecy;
* failure to seek help;
* lack of suicide knowledge and awareness among health professionals;
* suicide is a rare event.

The social stigma of suicide

In many cultures suicide is seen as shameful, sinful, weak, selfish or manipulative. These beliefs are held both by society as a whole as well as by those who experience suicidal thoughts. This acts to reinforce both secrecy and silence. Such beliefs may contribute to feelings of isolation, self-contempt and self-deprecation in individuals experiencing thoughts of suicide, and shame and guilt in those who have had loved ones who have committed suicide.

In some cultures self-inflicted death may be covertly sanctioned in specific sociocultural contexts, such as suicides committed in the name of family honour. In these circumstances silence, shame and secrecy may be attributed to both the act itself as well as the circumstances preceding the act.

In other situations, religious or secular authorities may overtly sanction suicide that is committed as an act of martyrdom. In these cases, public expression of self-inflicted death can be seen as a declaration of religious devotion, nationalistic expression or political belief.

Common suicide myths that serve to support and sustain the social stigma of suicide

Myth	Reality
If someone talks about suicide they are unlikely to actually do anything to harm themselves	Many people who die by suicide have communicated their feelings, thoughts or plans before their death
Suicide is always an impulsive act	Many people who commit suicide have experienced suicidal thoughts and have contemplated taking their own life before the act
Suicide is an expected or natural response to stress	Suicide is an abnormal outcome of stress. Everybody experiences stress... not everybody attempts suicide
Suicide is caused by stress	Suicide attempts or acts of self-harm may sometimes occur following an acute stressor (such as the breakup of a relationship or following an intense argument) but the event is a **behavioural trigger not a cause** of suicide
People who are **really** at risk for suicide are not ambivalent about completing the act	The intensity of suicidality waxes and wanes and many people who attempt or commit suicide struggle with their conviction to die
People who commit suicide are selfish and weak	Many people who commit suicide suffer from a mental disorder that may or may not have been recognized
Someone who is smart and successful would never commit suicide	Be careful... remember, suicidality is often kept secret. 'Suicide' has no cultural, ethnic, racial or socioeconomic boundaries
Talking about suicide with a depressed person will probably cause them to commit suicide	Many depressed people who have suicidal thoughts or plans are relieved when someone knows about them and is able to help them. Discussing suicidality with a depressed person **will not** lead them to commit suicide
There is nothing that can be done for a person who is suicidal	Many individuals who attempt suicide may be suffering from a mental disorder that will respond to appropriate and effective treatment. Appropriate treatment of a mental disorder significantly reduces the risk of suicide. For example, suicidality associated with depression usually resolves with effective treatment of the depressive disorder
People who attempt suicide are just looking for attention	In some people a suicide attempt is an event that leads to a first contact with a helping professional. **A desperate cry for help is not equivalent to wanting attention**

Failure to seek help

Many of those who commit suicide do not seek help and do not inform others of their plans. Moreover, many who are contemplating suicide or who are committed to completing suicide may not reveal their thoughts or plans even when directly asked. Thus, asking about suicidal ideation does not ensure that accurate or complete information will be received or that suicide will always be prevented. This, however, does not mean that health professionals should not conduct appropriate suicide assessments when known risk factors are present. In many cases such questioning will encourage the individual to share his or her thoughts and can be both a great relief and a reprieve from his or her sense of isolation. Indeed, empathic questioning of high-risk individuals about suicidal thoughts, intent or plans from a knowledgeable health professional will most often be seen as an expression of support, interest and professional competency. Such questioning can often encourage the suicidal individual to seek help when they otherwise would not.

Lack of suicide knowledge and awareness among health professionals

A common misconception among many health professionals is that talking to patients about suicide will increase the likelihood of the patient engaging in suicidal behaviours or committing suicide. This is not the case. Asking patients about suicidal thoughts will not plant or nurture these thoughts or wishes in the patient's mind. Rather, patients with suicidal thoughts often feel relieved that they have finally been given 'permission' to talk about these thoughts and feelings. Many patients who have suicidal ideation feel burdened, ashamed and/or sinful for having such thoughts. Some are frightened by these thoughts. Some interpret these thoughts as reinforcements for their own perceived worthlessness. Opening the door to open dialogue about such thoughts and fears may offer patients the opportunity to be heard and feel understood and may help alleviate patient psychological and emotional stress as well as potentially prevent suicide.

In fact, for those patients for whom suicide has become their 'only perceived option', disclosure may provide the opportunity to explore alternative choices that they could not see before.

Suicide is a rare event

Another issue that interferes with the prevention of completed suicide is the relative rarity of the event itself. As mentioned above, suicide attempts occur much more frequently than completed suicides (up to 20 times more frequently!) and suicidal ideation (having thoughts of wanting to die or of killing oneself) is more common still (up to six times more common than suicide attempts and up to 100 times more common than completed suicides!). Hence, many people who have suicidal thoughts and many of those who make a suicide attempt do not die from suicide.

Because suicide is a rare event, it is not considered useful to screen entire populations for suicidality or to routinely ask every single patient about suicidal ideas at every health professional contact. A number of risk factors, however, have been identified that can provide clinicians with a **risk profile** for suicide. Health professionals who are familiar with these risk factors can thereby identify potential 'at risk' patients for assessment of suicidality.

Can we always predict who will or who will not commit suicide?

Unfortunately, the answer is 'no'. What we can do is assess individual **'suicide risk'** based on identified **suicide risk and suicide protective factors** that may help identify those who are more or less likely to have a completed suicide in the near future. The health professional approaches the issue of suicide in the clinical setting by estimating the burden of risk. **How strong is the risk for suicide in the near future?** This is determined by learning how to identify and weigh both risk and protective factors and then formulating a clinical decision as to whether suicide risk is high, moderate or low.

Suicide: protective factors and risk factors

Identification of factors that may increase or decrease a patient's level of suicide risk can help clinicians to establish an estimate of the overall level of suicide risk for an individual patient, and this in turn can assist in the development of treatment plans that best address patient safety and target identified modifiable behavioural, psychosocial, environmental and personality factors.

It is important to remember, however, that not one protective or risk factor independently in and of itself can determine the event of suicide. Also, not all protective or risk factors are equally strong in prediction. For example, whereas gender is a risk factor (males are more likely to commit suicide than females in most countries studied), having a suicidal plan poses a much greater degree of risk than being male. When thinking about protective and risk factors for suicide it is important to think about these factors **in aggregate** and to view them within the context of the patient's experience. This will help you weigh how strong the risk will be for the individual you are dealing with.

Protective factors for suicide

Factors that are thought to protect the patient against suicide have been written about although the scientific data to support their notation are generally not very strong. They are listed below:

- absence of a mental disorder;
- employment;
- children in the home;
- sense of responsibility to family;
- pregnancy;
- strong religious beliefs;
- high life satisfaction;
- intact reality testing;
- positive coping skills;
- positive problem-solving skills;
- positive social support;
- positive therapeutic relationship.

> In the opinion of the authors of this manual, these factors have not been adequately demonstrated to prevent suicide. Thus, during an assessment of suicide risk in an individual, these should not be used to override those factors that identify suicide risk.

Risk factors for suicide

Risk factors for suicide will be considered under five headings noted below. The presence of one or more of these risk factors may increase an individual's risk for suicide but does not necessarily predict suicide. The recognition of risk factors can assist the health professional in identifying who may require a comprehensive assessment and in formulating the overall level of an individual's risk for suicide. The headings are:

1 Patient demographics: age and gender
2 Past and current suicidality
3 Psychiatric diagnosis and psychiatric symptoms
4 Individual history:
   - medical history
   - family history
   - psychosocial history
   - neurobiology
5 Personality strengths and weaknesses

Patient demographics: age and gender

Age and suicide

In North America, Western Europe (including the UK) and in most other countries for which data are available, suicide rates generally increase with increasing age. Projected on top of this trend are two peaks representing periods of increased risk. These periods correspond to two population groups: adolescents/young adults and the elderly.

In general, suicide rates rise sharply in late adolescence and early adulthood before levelling off through midlife and rising again after age 70. Among the 15 to 24-year-old age group, suicide rates in the USA tripled in the decades following the 1950s and became the third leading cause of death in young people. Contrary to popular opinion, the highest suicide rates in the first three decades of life are not in teenagers but in young adults. Over the past decade youth suicide has actually been decreasing in the USA, Canada and in many (but not all) other countries. Nonetheless, in many of these countries, suicide continues to be one of the three leading causes of death in young people between the ages of 15 and 24 years.

Question

What accounts for the rise in suicide rates during adolescence and young adulthood?

Answer

This increase parallels the rise in the incidence of mental illness. Many of the major mental disorders have their onset in adolescence. As severe mental disorders (depression, bipolar disorder, schizophrenia) increase so do suicide rates. Contrary to much popular opinion, suicide **is not** caused by the usual and expected stresses of adolescence! The vast majority of young people negotiate through their teens successfully.

The highest suicide rates are often found in the elderly. This may seem counterintuitive in the context of the epidemiological data on suicidal behaviours and self-destructive acts. Suicidal behaviours and suicide attempts are more common in the younger age groups than in the elderly. However, the suicidal behaviours that do occur in the elderly are more often likely to be lethal. Therefore, this second peak or rise in suicide rate after age 70 reflects a rise in completed suicides despite fewer overall attempts or self-destructive acts.

Question

What accounts for this rise in lethality of suicidal behaviours in the elderly?

Answer

There are a number of factors that may contribute to the higher rates of completed suicide in the elderly. In general, the elderly are less physically resilient, are more likely to be suffering from a variety of physical illnesses, are more likely to have access to medication that taken in excess or in combination have a greater likelihood of lethality. In many societies the elderly may be more isolated or experience greater poverty and, therefore, are less likely to be discovered or rescued following a suicide attempt than their younger counterparts. All of these factors reduce the likelihood of survival following a suicide attempt.

In addition, the elderly may be less likely to engage in impulsive suicidal behaviours and are more likely to have reached a definitive decision about ending their life by suicide after much contemplation and planning. Elders who commit suicide generally demonstrate a greater determination to die than younger individuals as evidenced by the fact that suicidal elders give fewer warnings signs of their ideas and plans; use more violent and potentially lethal methods to commit suicide; and engage in suicidal behaviours that involve greater planning and resolve.

Gender and suicide

The pattern of increasing suicide rates with increasing age is similar for both men and women, although rates in older adulthood are higher for men, which may be a reflection of higher rates of alcohol and/or substance abuse problems, which more often accompanies depression in men than in women.

Factors that may contribute to higher suicide rates in men compared with women include the following:

- Men are less likely to seek help for emotional or psychological problems than women.
- Men may be more behaviourally impulsive than women.
- Men tend to be less socially embedded than women.

- Men may be less willing to accept help for emotional or psychological problems than women.
- Men may choose more lethal suicide methods than women.

These gender differences provide women with a number of protective factors over their male counterparts. In addition to those outlined above, pregnancy and the presence of young children in the home are also suicide protective factors for women. It has been noted that women may attempt suicide or self-harm more frequently than men but that men are more likely to be successful if they make an attempt.

Question

Are there risk factors unique to women?

Answer

Female suicide is often associated with a social factor not usually found in male suicide – intimate partner (usually spousal) abuse. Both domestic sexual abuse and physical violence are associated with higher rates of female suicidal ideation and suicide attempts.

In some cultures the gender inequalities that women face, not only in civil society but also within the family, may increase their risk for suicide. Sociocultural and familial definitions and expectations of the female 'role' or position in family and society may also be a risk factor in individual cases. The value placed on female virtue and family honour must not be underestimated, particularly in societies or groups in which these ideals are strongly embedded. In such cases, actual or perceived transgression against these values can lead to social, spousal or family sanctions that are powerful enough to compel suicidal behaviour. For example, the high rates of suicide by poisoning in China and the self-harm/suicide by self-immolation (burning) in the Middle East may reflect these gender role issues.

Although pregnancy has been found to be a protective factor against suicide in women there is one exception – severe psychiatric illness following delivery (postpartum depression or postpartum psychosis) is associated with a higher risk of suicide as well as infanticide in women.

Postpartum depression

Fifty percent of women will experience symptoms including depressed mood, irritability, mood swings, crying spells, fatigue and anxiety following the delivery of a child. These symptoms usually occur within the first two weeks after giving birth and are referred to as the 'postpartum blues'. The postpartum blues are self-limiting, usually lasting several days, rarely more than a few weeks, and do not require medical intervention apart from reassurance and monitoring. The postpartum blues, however, may be a harbinger for a more serious problem, postpartum depression (PPD).

Postpartum depression affects up to 10–15% of women and usually develops within the first 4–6 weeks after childbirth. Women who experience PPD meet full criteria for a major depressive episode but tend to experience more mood fluctuation and more prominent anxiety symptoms compared with a non-postpartum-related depressive episode.

Mnemonic for symptoms of a depressive episode:
SAD A FACES
S – Sleep change
A – Appetite (weight change)
D – Dysphoria (low mood)
A – Anhedonia
F – Fatigue
A – Agitation/restlessness
C – Concentration
E – Esteem/guilt
S – Suicide

Some mothers with PPD demonstrate frank disinterest in the newborn or may become fearful of being left alone with the baby. Others may become preoccupied with the baby's wellbeing. This preoccupation may become obsessional and in some cases may reach delusional proportions. Mothers with PPD often experience feelings of intense shame, guilt, and incompetence in their role as care provider for their newborn, feelings that are often inadvertently reinforced by family, community and health-care providers who do not recognize the presence of an underlying disorder. Perinatal and postnatal support providers (i.e., physicians, nurses, midwives), community workers, and primary and pediatric care providers must be aware of the signs, symptoms and risk factors for PPD, and mothers experiencing symptoms of PPD must be evaluated. As with depression itself, PPD is associated with an increased risk of suicide, and may be associated with neglect of the newborn and in severe cases (particularly when associated with psychosis) infanticide.

Postpartum psychosis

Postpartum psychosis (PPP) is estimated to occur in 1 per 1000 childbirths. This disorder is believed to be closely associated with the mood disorders (bipolar and major depressive disorder). Approximately 50% of women who experience PPP have a family history of mood disorder. Some 50–60% of women affected are primiparous (first delivery) and many (50%) have a history of perinatal (delivery) complications.

The first symptoms of PPP usually begin within the first 2 weeks following delivery. Many of the initial symptoms of PPP may be reminiscent of the postpartum blues: depressed mood, irritability, mood swings, crying spells, fatigue and anxiety. In the early stages of the illness, before the onset of frank psychosis, these symptoms are often accompanied by agitation and insomnia. Later, symptoms such as suspiciousness, cognitive deficits (confusion and incoherence), and obsessive concern about the baby's health and welfare may develop. Many women with PPP develop delusional beliefs involving the child: beliefs that the child is possessed or evil; that the child is dead; or that the child is defective. Some mothers may deny the pregnancy and birth; fear or loathe the child; and have impulses to harm the child. Persecutory and somatic delusions are also common. In addition, women with PPP may develop hallucinations that may include command-type auditory hallucinations telling the mother to harm herself and/or the baby and other children in the home. Approximately 5% of mothers affected by PPP are believed to commit suicide and up to 4% commit infanticide.

Summary of risk factors associated with age and gender

Age and gender	Higher risk	Lower risk
Age	Elderly 15–35 years	Prepubertal
Gender	Male	Female
Women	Intimate partner abuse Domestic abuse Postpartum depression Postpartum psychosis Rigid role expectations Institutionalized gender inequality	Pregnancy Young children in the home

Past and current suicidality
Past history of suicide attempts

Past suicidal behaviours are a major risk factor for suicide. In many published studies, up to 50% of those who die by suicide have made at least one previous attempt. Suicide attempts are 10–20 times more prevalent than suicide; therefore, most individuals who make a suicide attempt will not die by suicide. Identification of factors that increase an individual's likelihood for suicide following an attempt can aid the clinician in estimating suicide risk. Factors that increase the risk of death by suicide in patients who have made a past attempt include the presence of a longstanding medical illness or psychiatric condition (particularly depression or alcohol abuse), social isolation and poor social supports. In addition, there are a number of features of past suicide attempts that make future suicide more likely. Past suicide attempts that were serious in nature (i.e., those leading to serious adverse consequences such as medical disability), those involving high intent and use of highly lethal methods (firearm or hanging), and those that were premeditated with measures taken to avoid discovery are associated with an increased risk for future suicide.

   Characteristics of past attempts that increase future suicide risk include:
* presence of a longstanding medical illness;
* presence of psychiatric illness;
* low levels of social cohesion;
* serious attempt with adverse consequences;
* high intent;
* use of highly lethal means;
* measures taken to avoid discovery.

Summary of past suicide behaviour risk factors

Past suicidal behaviours associated with increased suicide risk	Higher risk	Lower risk
Detected suicide attempts	Multiple attempts	First attempt
Undetected suicide attempts	Planned	Impulsive
Aborted suicide attempts	Low likelihood of rescue	High likelihood of
Self-harming behaviours	High intent	rescue
	Use of highly lethal method	Ambivalence
	Availability of lethal means	Low intent
	Serious medical consequences	Low lethal method

Current suicidal ideation, intent and plans

The presence of suicidal ideation is associated with a higher risk for suicide. As mentioned above, the vast majority of individuals with suicidal ideation will not die by suicide and some individuals who do commit suicide may not reveal their suicidal thoughts even when directly asked. Notwithstanding, clinicians must ask any patient who expresses depression or hopelessness, about the presence and nature of suicidal thoughts, the presence of a suicidal plan, as well as the intent and commitment to follow through with suicidal plans in order to estimate the individual's risk for suicide.

Suicidal ideation

Suicidal ideation refers to thoughts, fantasies, ruminations and preoccupations about death, self-harm and self-inflicted death. The greater the magnitude and persistence of the suicidal thoughts the higher is the risk for eventual suicide.

Suicidal intent

Suicidal intent refers to the patient's expectation and commitment to die by suicide. The strength of the patient's intent to die may be reflected in the patient's subjective belief in the lethality of the chosen method, which may be more relevant than the chosen method's objective lethality.

For example:

A patient who ingests a bottle of medicine 'A' (a medicine that is known by pharmacists and health professionals not to cause death in overdose) and who absolutely believes that ingesting that quantity of medicine 'A' will be lethal is demonstrating high intent even though the medicine chosen is unlikely to lead to death.

The stronger the **intent to die** the greater the risk for completed suicide.

Suicidal plan

The more detailed and specific the suicide plan the greater the level of suicide risk. Particular attention should be paid to the chosen method of harm (particularly its lethality), the chosen timing and setting of the event, the accessibility of the method chosen, and actions taken by the patient to prepare for the event. In general, suicide plans that are premeditated and well thought-out (writing a suicide note, preparing a will, giving away personal belongings or property, actions taken to secure or ensure access to means or method of suicide), involve a highly lethal method (firearm or hanging), and are planned in a setting and at a time when discovery is unlikely are indicative of high risk for suicide.

The suicidal method chosen is a significant factor in determining risk of death by suicide. The more lethal the method the more likely the individual is of dying from suicide. In many Western countries guns and jumping from heights are the lethal means chosen. Globally, the most common methods of suicide are ingestion of pesticides, the use of firearms, and medication overdose. Among women in India and the Middle East self-immolation is increasingly being recognized as a means for suicide.

Question

Are there specific aspects of a suicide plan that may be associated with higher lethality?

Answer

Important aspects of a suicide plan that are suggestive of the plan's potential lethality include: the chosen method; availability of means; the individual's understanding and belief about the lethality of the chosen method; the chance of rescue; steps taken to enact the plan; and the individual's preparedness for death.

- **Method**: the choice of a higher lethality method is associated with higher suicide risk (i.e., firearms, jumping from heights, pesticide ingestion and motor vehicle accidents). Firearms, poisoning, hanging and drug ingestion are the most commonly used methods for suicide.
- **Availability of means**: for example, access to a firearm or access to liquid pesticide.
- **Patient's belief about the lethality of the method:** suggestive of patient's intent and commitment to die by self-inflicted harm.
- **Chance of rescue:** low chance of rescue associated with higher risk of successful suicide.

- **Steps taken to enact plan:** actions taken to carry out the plan such as purchasing of a firearm, hoarding pills, establishing date, time and setting for the event, ensuring isolation and low risk of discovery all increase suicide risk.
- **Preparedness for death:** plans made by patients to set their affairs in order may be indicative of anticipated death by suicide (i.e., plans made to fulfil financial obligations, making of a will, discarding possessions, writing letters to loved ones, making amends with others, and formulating a suicide note).

Summary of suicidality risk factors

Suicidality associated with increased suicide risk	Higher risk	Lower risk
Suicidal ideation	Frequent Intense Prolonged	Infrequent Low intensity Transient
Suicidal intent	High	Low
Suicidal plans	Premeditated Well-planned Highly lethal means Access to means	No plan Choice of low lethality No access to means

Psychiatric symptoms and diagnosis

Psychiatric disorder is the strongest attributable risk factor for suicide. Psychiatric disorders with the highest associated risk include the mood disorders, psychotic disorders, anxiety disorders, some of the personality disorders as well as substance abuse and dependence (particularly alcohol).

In addition, specific psychiatric symptoms, within or outside of the context of a psychiatric disorder, have been associated with increased suicide risk.

Psychiatric symptoms

Psychiatric symptoms associated with increased suicide risk include:

- depression
- severe anxiety
- panic attacks
- hopelessness

- command hallucinations
- impulsivity
- aggression
- severe anhedonia
  Other psychiatric symptoms that may increase suicide risk are:
- dysphoria
- shame or humiliation
- decreased self-esteem
- violence toward others
- agitation
- akathisia/restlessness
- anger
- insomnia

Summary of psychiatric symptoms that may increase suicide risk

Psychiatric symptoms associated with increased suicide risk	Higher risk	Lower risk
Psychosis	Hopelessness	Optimism
Depression/dysphoria	Severe anhedonia	Religiosity
Hopelessness	Severe anxiety	High life satisfaction
Anxiety	Panic attacks	
Panic attacks		
Shame or humiliation		
Decreased self-esteem		
Impulsiveness		
Aggression		
Agitation		
Akathisia/restlessness		

Before beginning a discussion of the risk factors associated with the different disorders, let us take a look at risk factors that have been associated with increased risk of suicide independent of diagnosis. A higher risk for suicide may apply to individuals suffering from a psychiatric illness who are also socially isolated; who have experienced significant personal, academic, vocational or financial loss; who have maladaptive coping skills; and those who have, as a consequence of their illness, become dependent on others, or have lost previously held skills, social status or familial role. In addition, the presence of depressive symptoms, hopelessness, or associated alcohol or other substance use disorder may increase risk when found concurrently with any psychiatric disorder.

Factors that may increase suicide risk in individuals with any psychiatric disorder are:

- social isolation;
- loss of family role/status;

- interpersonal losses;
- vocational/occupational loss;
- loss of previous skills/competencies;
- awareness of deficits with recovery;
- substance or alcohol abuse/dependence;
- poor problem-solving capacity (cognitive impairment);
- depressive symptoms;
- hopelessness.

Psychiatric diagnosis

Psychiatric disorders associated with increased suicide risk include the following:

1 Mood disorders
2 Psychotic disorders
3 Anxiety disorders
4 Alcohol and other substance use disorders
5 Personality disorders

Mood disorders

In many reported studies it has been noted that about 50% of people who die by suicide may suffer from a major depressive disorder. Mood disorders confer a 20-fold increased risk of death by suicide. Major depressive disorder and the depressive and mixed phases of bipolar disorder are the diagnoses most often found in suicide deaths. For younger patients suffering from major depressive disorder or bipolar disorder, suicides are more likely to occur early in the illness course particularly if depressive symptoms are accompanied by panic attacks, severe anxiety, diminished concentration, severe insomnia, alcohol abuse, and anhedonia (loss of pleasure or interest in previously enjoyed activities). The presence of hopelessness, ranging from pessimism and negative expectation about the future to despairing about the future, has also been associated with increased suicide risk particularly in later stages of the illness. Individuals who are experiencing a depressive episode within the context of a bipolar illness (a bipolar depression) may be at an even higher risk of suicide than those who have depression outside the context of a bipolar illness (unipolar depression).

Clinical depression – in DSM (*Diagnostic and Statistical Manual of Mental Disorders*) terminology often referred to as major depressive disorder and dysthymia – is a common psychiatric illness that affects up to 6–8% of the population. It is not to be confused with depressive symptoms that manifest themselves in the context of unhappy life events that may more reasonably be considered to be a natural part of human existence. Clinical depression (to which the term depression used in this manual refers) tends to have an initial onset in adolescence or early adulthood and is highly correlated to the increased suicide rates that occur during this time. It is a chronic episodic illness with the great majority of individuals experiencing a further episode within five years of the onset of the first. Although depression runs in families and recent research has demonstrated genetic propensities to depression, suicidal behaviour in depression is the output of a complex interplay between illness and environmental factors. When depression occurs concurrently with a chronic medical condition (such as pain or heart disease) or a life-threatening medical disorder (such as cancer) suicide risk may be substantially increased.

By convention, clinical depression is diagnosed following syndromal criteria spelled out in one of two diagnostic classification systems: the DSM or the ICD (*International Classification of Disease*). In general, individuals must demonstrate most of the following symptoms, which are different than their usual mood state, have persisted over time and have led to functional impairment:

* depressed mood;
* loss of interest or pleasure;
* lack of energy;
* difficulty in concentration;
* loss of appetite;
* thoughts and feelings of worthlessness or hopelessness;
* guilty ruminations;
* pronounced sleep difficulties;
* suicidal ideation/plans (or the feeling that life is not worth living).

The individual experiences significant difficulties in self-motivation across many life domains (interpersonal, social, vocational) as a result of the low mood and negative cognitions. In many cases (and in many cultures) somatic symptoms such as difficulty in sleeping, headaches, lack of energy, etc. may be the most common presentation of depression. Health professionals should be aware of this presentation and screen for the presence of depressed mood or depressive cognitions (such as worthlessness, hopelessness and lack of pleasure) when individuals present with such complaints.

High levels of hopelessness alone, with or without a diagnosis of depression, have been associated with an increased likelihood of suicidal behaviours.

Every depressed patient should have ongoing monitoring of suicide risk – even when they are 'feeling better' or 'getting well'. This is particularly important during the period early in treatment as initial improvements in energy or behavioural side effects of some medications may increase risk of suicidal thoughts or self-harm behaviours.

In addition to the diagnosis itself, the presence of specific symptoms occurring within the depressive syndrome may be associated with increased suicide risk. These include:

* hopelessness
* panic attacks
* severe anxiety
* severe anhedonia
* psychosis

Psychotic disorders

The presence of psychosis contributes to more than 10% of suicides, and schizophrenia is associated with a tenfold increased risk of death by suicide. Studies have shown that up to 50% of schizophrenia patients may attempt suicide at some point in the course of their illness. Suicide attempts in schizophrenia are frequently precipitated by depression, psychosocial stressors and psychotic symptoms; are often medically serious; and are often associated with a high degree of intent.

Suicide in schizophrenia is most common during the early years following illness onset, and an increased risk of suicide has been correlated with a number of factors including patient attributes, symptom characteristics, as well as period in illness course. Patients at higher risk for suicide include those who have a chronic illness course, those who have required multiple psychiatric hospitalizations and those who have made a previous suicide attempt. In addition, patients with significant depressive symptoms, patients with good premorbid functioning and those who understand, or have insight into the implications of having a chronic psychotic illness (those who appreciate the negative impact of the illness on their personal, social and vocational functioning and achievement, and those who recognize a loss of previous skills and competencies) are also at high risk, particularly if they are pessimistic about the benefits of treatment. Other factors associated with increased suicide risk include male gender, younger age, social isolation, severe agitation or akathisia, and the presence of prominent positive psychotic symptoms. Patients who feel terrorized by their symptoms, those experiencing persecutory delusions and those experiencing aggressive or suicidal command hallucinations may be at particularly high risk for self-injurious behaviours and completed suicide (the presence of prominent negative psychotic symptoms, such as apathy and avolition, is associated with a reduced risk of suicide).

Command hallucinations are auditory hallucinations that instruct the individual to perform specific actions, think specific thoughts, or behave in specific ways. Not all command-type hallucinations necessarily pose a safety issue for the patient. For example, command hallucinations that instruct the patient to close a door or wear a particular colour of clothing are benign (although they may be distressing to the patient). On the other hand, command hallucinations that instruct the patient to engage in risk-taking behaviours, to harm themselves or to harm others, may be lethal!

It is difficult to predict which patients are more or less likely to obey command hallucinations; thus, any patient who is experiencing dangerous command hallucinations should be closely monitored.

Patient variables that have been associated with a higher likelihood of patient compliance with hallucinatory commands include the following:
- Patients who are able to identify the hallucinatory voice.
- Patients who are experiencing a severe psychotic disturbance.
- Patients experiencing less dangerous commands.
- Patients with new-onset command hallucinations.
- Patients experiencing command hallucinations outside of a hospital environment.

For many patients the period immediately following discharge from hospital and during periods of improvement after relapse confer the highest risk for suicide or suicide attempts. This may be partly attributable to the improved insight that often accompanies symptom improvement, which may allow patients to appreciate: the impact of the illness on their ability to function in and be accepted by society; the loss of previous skills, relationships and social position; and the consequences of the stigmatization of and discrimination against the mentally ill. In addition, the onset of postpsychotic depression following an acute episode has been identified as a vulnerable time for schizophrenia patients, particularly young males with good insight and good premorbid functioning.

Factors that may increase suicide risk in schizophrenia include:
- Insight into deficits caused by illness.
- Self-harm/violent command hallucinations.
- Akathisia – may be related to side effects of antipsychotic medications.
- Agitation – may be related to side effects of antipsychotic medications.
- Depressive symptoms.
- Feelings of hopelessness.
- Unemployment.
- Recent hospital discharge.
- Social isolation.
- Male gender.
- Age less than 45 years.

Anxiety disorders
Suicidal ideation and suicide attempts are common in individuals with anxiety disorders. Anxiety disorders may play a role in 15–20% of suicides and confer a 6–10% increase in suicide risk, particularly if associated with panic attacks, depression and/or alcohol use. The presence of severe anxiety or panic attacks, within or outside the context of an anxiety disorder, have themselves been associated with higher risk for suicide.

Alcohol and substance use disorders

Alcohol abuse or dependence may play a role in 25–50% of deaths by suicide and is associated with a sixfold increased suicide mortality rate compared with the general population and a lifetime risk for suicide of up to 15%. Substance abuse, including polysubstance abuse, may also be a common precursor to suicide. In contrast to depression and schizophrenia, suicide among substance abusers often occurs late in the disease course after the chronic effects of the disorder have heavily impacted on health, social, interpersonal, economic and vocational/occupational functioning. In addition to being at higher risk for completed suicide, patients with substance use disorders, particularly alcohol abuse or dependence, are at high risk for self-inflicted harm and suicide attempts.

Alcohol abuse in the context of a psychiatric disorder is an important risk factor for suicide. Major depressive episodes can be identified in up to three-quarters of alcoholics who die by suicide. Risk for suicide among patients with alcohol use disorders is increased in both males and females, but as with suicide generally, the rate of completed suicide is higher in men and the rate of suicide attempts is greater in women.

Substance use disorders: additional risk factors for suicide

- Recent or impending interpersonal loss.
- Presence of other psychiatric disorders.
- Loss or disruption of a close interpersonal relationship.
- Threatened loss of a relationship.
- Presence of a depressive episode.

Alcohol use disorders: additional risk factors for suicide

- Communications of suicidal intent.
- Previous suicide attempts.
- Continued or heavier drinking.
- Recent unemployment.
- Living alone.
- Poor social support.
- Legal difficulties.
- Financial difficulties.
- Serious medical illness.
- Other psychiatric disorders.
- Personality disturbance.
- Other substance use.

Question

Can alcohol intoxication itself be a risk factor for suicide even if the person does not have alcohol abuse or dependence?

Answer

Alcohol intoxication itself, even in the absence of alcohol abuse or dependence, may be a risk factor for suicide. A significant proportion of those who die by suicide are found to have ingested alcohol before their attempt. Those who consume alcohol before committing suicide may be more likely to be experiencing an interpersonal or other psychosocial stressor and less likely to have sought help before death. Suicide in the context of alcohol intoxication may more likely be impulsive rather than planned and may be more likely to involve a highly lethal method such as a firearm.

Personality disorders

According to a number of studies, having a personality disorder, particularly a borderline or antisocial personality disorder, may be a factor in up to 5% of suicides. Lifetime rates of suicide for these disorders range from 3% to 9%. Rates of self-harm behaviours and suicide attempts are high in this patient population.

Personality disorders: additional risk factors for completed suicide:

- Unemployment.
- Financial difficulty.
- Family discord.
- Interpersonal conflicts.
- Loss.
- Impulsivity.

Summary of risk factors associated with psychiatric diagnosis

Psychiatric disorders associated with increased suicide risk	Higher risk	Lower risk
Major depressive disorder	Hopelessness	Absence of acute episode of
Bipolar disorder (depressive or	Severe depression	mental disorder
mixed episode)	Acute psychosis	Treated mental illness
Schizophrenia	Substance abuse	Supportive environment
Substance use disorder	Noncompliance	Compliant with treatment
Personality disorders	Poorly controlled	Low substance use
(particularly borderline	symptoms	
personality disorder)		

Individual history

Medical history

Physical illness may increase suicide risk, particularly if the condition is associated with functional impairments, cognitive impairment, pain, disfigurement, increased dependence on others, and decreases in vision or hearing. Neurological disorders such as epilepsy, multiple sclerosis, Huntington disease, and brain and spinal cord injury are associated with a particularly high risk for suicide.

Other physical disorders that have been found to be associated with an increased risk for suicide include:
* Human immunodeficiency virus (HIV)/acquired immunodeficiency syndrome (AIDS).
* Malignancies.
* Peptic ulcer disease.
* Systemic lupus erythematosus.
* Chronic hemodialysis-treated renal failure.
* Heart disease.
* Chronic obstructive pulmonary disease.
* Prostate disease.

The risk for suicide or suicide attempts in the context of physical illness is highly correlated with the presence of a psychiatric illness (particularly depression) or psychiatric symptoms (such as hopelessness) as well as the individual patient's personality and coping style, availability of social supports, presence of psychosocial stressors, previous history of suicidal behaviours, and the meaning and consequences of the illness to the patient. In the elderly, the onset of dementia may increase suicide risk.

Although rates of depression are increased in those with serious medical illness depression is not a logical or expected outcome of having a chronic or life-threatening disease (most people with chronic or life-threatening diseases may have depressed or despondent feelings but most people will not develop clinical depression). When clinical depression does occur in a person with a chronic or life-threatening disease, it must be appropriately treated and the individual must be evaluated for suicidal ideas, intentions and plans. Depression and associated suicidal ideation tend to be underdetected and undertreated in the medically ill.

Characteristics of a medical disorder associated with higher suicide risk:
* Chronic disease.
* Neurological disorder associated with:
  - pain;
  - functional impairment;
  - cognitive impairment;
  - loss of sight or hearing;
  - disfigurement;
  - increased dependence on others.
* Presence of a psychiatric disorder.

- Presence of psychiatric symptoms.

Increased suicidality in HIV/AIDS may be associated with the following:
- Presence of HIV dementia (often characterized by labile mood, behavioural disinhibition, impaired judgment, impulsivity).
- Presence of a psychiatric disorder.
- Substance abuse.
- Previous suicide attempts.
- Depression.
- Greater number of disease symptoms.
- Loneliness.
- Need for support.
- Younger age.
- Current stressors (unemployment, bereavement, etc.).
- Poor adaptive functioning.
- Hopelessness.
- Internalizing pattern.

Summary of medical history risk factors

Medical disorders associated with increased risk	Higher risk	Lower risk
Neurological disorder	Chronic illness	Disease remission
HIV/AIDS	Pain	Feels physically well
Malignancies	Functional impairment	
Peptic ulcer disease	Loss of sight or hearing	
Systemic lupus erythematosus	Disfigurement	
Chronic hemodialysis-treated renal failure	Increased dependence on others	
Heart disease		
Chronic obstructive pulmonary disease		
Prostate disease		

Family history

A number of factors in the family history influence the risk for suicidal behaviours and completed suicide. Both a history of suicide (particularly in first-degree relatives) and a history of psychiatric illness in the family confer increased risk. In addition, family violence, abuse or neglect may be associated with higher risk.

Genetic factors may also play a role. Monozygotic (identical) twins have a significantly higher rate of both completed suicide and suicide attempts than do dizygotic (nonidentical or fraternal) twins. Adoption studies that have followed children who have been raised by their biological families and compared them with adopted-away children raised by adoptive families have shown that suicide rates of adopted-away children are comparable with those of their biological families rather than their adopted families.

There may be genetic factors that are specific to suicide that might not be the same as those that are associated with psychiatric illnesses (see 'Neurobiology of suicide' below).

Summary of family history risk factors

Family history associated with increased suicide risk	Higher risk	Lower risk
Suicide	Suicide in first-degree	No family history of suicide
Mental disorder	relative	No family history of mental
	Mental illness in first-degree relative	illness

Psychosocial history
The presence or absence of social and emotional supports plays an important part in the estimation of suicide risk. Whereas the presence of a strong social support system may reduce suicide risk the absence of a support system, living alone and social isolation can increase the risk for suicide. The presence and involvement of family, friends and meaningful others in the individual's life has a powerful protective influence in terms of both risk for completed suicide as well as suicide attempts.

Question

Does sexual orientation or choice of intimate partner influence suicide risk?

Answer

There are insufficient numbers of appropriately controlled studies currently available to specifically answer this question. However, studies involving diverse populations do suggest that homosexual or bisexual individuals are at higher risk for suicide attempts particularly among younger age groups. Suicide risk factors for this group may include cultural attitudes, stigma and discrimination against gays and lesbians, stress related to disclosure of sexual orientation to friends and family, gender nonconformity, and aggression against homosexuals. If teenagers who are struggling with issues of homosexuality become concurrently clinically depressed they may be at higher risk for a suicide attempt.

Question

Does marital status influence suicide risk?

Answer

Being married may be protective against suicide although the nature of the marital relationship must be considered. Conflictive or abusive marriages may be more likely to have a higher rather than a lower risk for suicide. Notwithstanding this, the suicide rate among single adults is twice that of married adults, and rates among those who are divorced, separated, or widowed are four to five times higher than those for married individuals. However, it is not possible to determine if this is a cause-and-effect relationship. Are people who are less prone to suicide able to create and hold long-term intimate relationships or does the presence of a long-term intimate relationship mitigate suicide, or both?

Question

Does employment status affect suicide risk?

Answer

Unemployment, and financial and legal difficulties have been associated with increased suicide risk. For some individuals, unemployment may be associated with a number of other factors that may increase suicide risk. For example, loss of employment may translate into loss of financial and family security, loss of residence, and significant interpersonal, marital and emotional stress. Alternatively, unemployment, job loss or failure to gain and maintain employment may reflect loss of previous competencies as a consequence of a physical or psychiatric disorder; maladaptive personality traits that are disruptive to the workplace or interfere with working with others; psychosocial circumstances including poverty, discrimination, lack of schooling or vocational training; or adverse childhood experiences. Thus the relationship between unemployment and suicidality may be bidirectional.

Question

Does the type of employment influence suicide risk?

Answer

Health-care professionals, particularly physicians and dentists, appear to be at higher risk of suicide compared with other professional groups. The reason for this is unknown.

Question

Does current or past abuse influence suicide risk?

Answer

Suicide rates are increased at least tenfold in those with a history of childhood sexual or physical abuse. Suicide rates are also higher in those exposed to domestic partner abuse. The risk for suicide attempts in individuals who have experienced recent domestic partner violence is four- to eight-fold higher than the risk for individuals without such experiences.

Question

Do cultural and religious beliefs influence suicide risk?

Answer

Beliefs about life, death and the afterlife are heavily influenced by culture, religion and society. Attitudes and beliefs about death and suicide held by different cultural and subcultural groups can significantly influence the rate of both completed suicide and suicide attempts. Cultures that overtly or covertly condone suicide as an acceptable way to deal with shame, humiliation, physical illness or distress are less prohibitive of suicide than cultures that view suicide as a sinful or criminal act. Thus, an understanding of an individual's sociocultural and religious beliefs regarding death and suicide are important when estimating individual suicide risk. For example, for individuals with strong religious beliefs who ascribe to a faith that prohibits suicide, religious conviction may be a protective factor against suicide. On the other hand, for an individual who ascribes to a culture in which suicide is an accepted traditional approach to familial or personal shame, the failure of a marriage or the loss of social position may place that individual at high risk for suicide.

Other cultures may overtly sanction suicide committed as an act of martyrdom, such as self-inflicted death committed as a declaration of religious devotion, nationalism or political belief.

Question

What about having hope or being able to identify reasons for living?

Answer

The ability of the individual to identify 'reasons for living' may be a protective factor against suicide. For one, it argues against 'hopelessness' and 'pessimism' by focusing individuals on what they have in their lives and promoting feelings of optimism. The presence of young children in the home, pregnancy, and a sense of responsibility to family are some of the protective 'reasons for living' cited by individuals with suicidal ideation.

Summary of psychosocial history risk factors

Psychosocial history associated with increased suicide risk	Higher risk	Lower risk
Lack of social support	Divorced or widowed	Married
Unemployment	Unemployed	Employment
Drop in socioeconomic status	Conflictual interpersonal relationships	Stable relationships
Family discord	Low personal achievement	Children in the home
Domestic violence	Social isolation	Good achievement
Recent stressful life event	Poor interpersonal relationships	Positive social support
Childhood sexual/physical abuse	Domestic violence	Positive therapeutic relationship
	Sexual abuse	Supportive family
	Physical abuse	Absence of abuse

Neurobiology of suicide

In addition to the genetic evidence from twin studies for suicide cited earlier, a number of biological factors associated with suicide have been identified. For example, neurobiological studies have found reduced levels of serotonin metabolites (5-hydroxyindoleacetic acid) in the CNS fluid of adult suicide victims. Serotonin is a brain neurochemical implicated in the regulation of mood and cognition. Abnormalities of brain serotonin function have been demonstrated in patients who suffer from a variety of psychiatric illnesses, most notably depression. More recently, increases in the numbers of brain serotonin receptor 2A (5-HT$_{2A}$) and genetic abnormalities of the serotonin system (polymorphism of the serotonin 2 receptor gene) have been described. These seem to be independent of the serotonin abnormalities found in depression without suicide.

Studies have also suggested an alteration in the hypothalamic–pituitary–adrenal axis in individuals at risk for suicide and in the growth hormone response to the chemical apomorphine. Additionally, research into neurotrophins, which are molecules that are important in brain synaptic plasticity and in the maintenance and growth of nerve cells, has identified abnormalities in a number of these compounds – such as brain-derived neurotrophic factor (BDNF), neurotrophin 3 (NT-3) and nerve growth factor (NGF) – in specific brain regions (the hippocampus and the prefrontal cortex) in successful suicides. In addition, gene expression studies of postmortem brain tissue suggest biological differences in those who commit suicide even when controlling for the presence of a depressive disorder.

Taken as a whole these studies suggest that there is a relationship between the neurotransmitter systems involved in depression and suicide but that individuals who commit suicide may have additional underlying genetic vulnerabilities that increase their risk. This research is still in its infancy and it is not currently possible to identify which individuals may carry this enhanced genetic risk. In the future, though, neurobiology may prove to be one of the most important risk factors for suicide.

Personality strengths and weaknesses

There is no such thing as a 'suicidal' personality. However, a patient's individual personality traits, ability to manage emotional and psychological pain, problem-solving skills, past responses to stress, and their ability to use internal and external resources during crises are important factors that may mitigate or increase the risk for suicide. Individuals who lack healthy coping strategies to deal with life adversity may be at higher risk for suicide. Healthy and well-developed coping skills help buffer stressful life events and allow individuals to access internal and external resources during crises.

In terms of personality, suicide risk may be associated with hostile, helpless, dependent and rigid personality traits. Individuals at higher risk of suicide may include those with rigid 'all or none' thinking. These individuals often have difficulty in problem solving during times of stress. Even if they are ambivalent about suicide they may see suicide as their only option because they are unable to come up with alternative strategies. In addition, individuals who are perfectionistic with excessively high personal expectations, may be at higher risk for suicide particularly in the context of perceived failure or humiliation. Individuals who have an enduring hopeless, fatalistic or pessimistic approach to life may also be at higher risk.

Summary of personality risk factors

Personality features associated with increased suicide risk	Higher risk	Lower risk
Lack of coping skills	Poor insight	Insightful
Lack of problem-solving skills	Rigid thinking	Sense of responsibility to family
Pessimism	Poor affective	Good reality testing
Hopelessness	control	Positive coping skills
Perfectionism	Manipulative	Positive problem-solving skills
Rigid or black-and-white thinking		Flexible
		Able to manage emotion/affect

By knowing these risk factors will I be able to prevent all patients from committing suicide?

Unfortunately, the answer is 'no'. No specific risk factor or set of risk factors has been identified that is consistently predictive of suicide or other suicidal behaviours.

Identification of 'suicide risk factors' does not allow a completely accurate prediction of when or if a specific individual will in fact die by suicide. Thus, suicide assessment scales that rely on the cataloging of patient risk factors, although a useful clinical aid in the assessment of suicide risk, cannot by themselves be used successfully to predict who will commit suicide. They can, however, give the clinician an idea of how significant the total risk load may be and thus flag those individuals for whom preventive interventions should be immediately initiated. Thus, a scale such as the Tool for Assessment of Suicide Risk (TASR), which is described later in this manual, can be a useful tool in the clinical evaluation of patients. Additionally, risk factors when taken together to identify the 'burden' of risk are most useful in addressing proximal rather than distal events. Accurately predicting the future is difficult enough. Accurately predicting the distant future may not be possible.

What can be done?

Remember… most patients who experience suicidal thoughts or engage in suicide behaviours will not die by suicide. Most will choose life rather than death.

As discussed in the introduction, suicide is complex and is influenced by innumerable underlying factors. Some of these factors will respond to appropriately targeted interventions. This is particularly true of those individuals who may be suffering from a mental disorder. Health professionals can ensure that each patient receives a thorough clinical evaluation with attention given to the patient's current presentation, individual strengths and weaknesses, history and psychosocial situation. This information can then be used to estimate the patient's suicide risk with the primary goal of reducing that risk and thereby reducing the likelihood of death by suicide. Identification and treatment of an existing mental disorder, for example, can significantly reduce individual suicide risk.

Summary of suicide risk factors

Areas of assessment	Higher risk	Lower risk
Age		
Youth	Elderly	Prepubertal
Adult	15–35 years	
Elderly		
Gender		
Male	Male	Female
Female		
Suicidality		
Suicidal ideation		
Suicidal plans	Frequent	Infrequent
Suicide intent	Intense	Low intensity
Suicide attempts	Prolonged	Transient
Lethality of chosen method		
Past suicidal behaviour		
Past attempts/self-harm	Multiple attempts	First attempt
Nature and severity of past	Planned attempts	Impulsive attempts
suicidal behaviours	Low likelihood of rescue	High likelihood of
Context of suicidal	High intent	rescue
behaviours	Use of highly lethal method	Ambivalence
Intent of past behaviours	Availability of means	Low intent
Feelings about past suicidal		Low lethal method
behaviours		

Continued

Areas of assessment	Higher risk	Lower risk
Psychiatric history		
Major depressive disorder	Severe depression	Absence of mental
Bipolar disorder (depressive	Acute psychosis	disorder
or mixed episode)	Substance abuse	Treated mental illness
Schizophrenia	Severe personality disorder	Mild depression
Alcohol use disorder	Noncompliance	Well controlled
Personality disorders	Poorly controlled	Compliant with
(particularly borderline		treatment
personality disorder)		Low substance use
Cognitive impairment		
Psychiatric symptoms		
Psychosis	Hopelessness	Optimism
Depression/dysphoria	Severe anhedonia	Religiosity
Hopelessness	Severe anxiety	Life satisfaction
Severe anxiety	Panic attacks	
Panic attacks		
Shame or humiliation		
Decreased self-esteem		
Impulsiveness		
Aggression		
Agitation		
Psychosocial history		
Lack of social support	Divorced or widowed	Married
Unemployment	Unemployed	Employment
Drop in socioeconomic	Conflictual interpersonal	Stable relationships
status	relationships	Children in the home
Family discord	Low achievement	Good achievement
Domestic violence	Social isolation	Positive social support
Recent stressful life event	Poor interpersonal	Positive therapeutic
Childhood sexual/physical	relationships	relationship
abuse	Domestic violence	Supportive family
	Sexual abuse	Absence of abuse
	Physical abuse	

Continued

Areas of assessment	Higher risk	Lower risk
Medical history		
Neurological disorder	Chronic illness	Healthy
HIV/AIDS	Associated pain	Feels physically well
Malignancies	Functional impairment	Pregnancy
Peptic ulcer disease	Loss of sight or hearing	
Systemic lupus	Disfigurement	
erythematosus	Increased dependence on	
Chronic hemodialysis-	others	
treated renal failure		
Heart disease		
Chronic obstructive		
pulmonary disease		
Prostate disease		
Family history		
Suicide	Suicide in first-degree relative	No family history of
Mental disorder	First-degree relative with	suicide
	mental illness	No family history of
		mental illness
Personality features		
Lack of coping skills	Poor insight	Insightful
Lack of problem-solving	Rigid thinking	Sense of responsibility
skills	Poor affective control	to family
Pessimism		Good reality testing
Hopelessness		ability
Perfectionism		Positive coping skills
Rigid or black-and-white		Positive problem-
thinking		solving skills
		Flexible
		Able to manage
		emotion/affect

Chapter 2
Suicide Risk Assessment

This next section of the manual will take you through the process of assessing suicide risk. It uses the information already presented in the manual and assists you in applying it in the clinical situation. The Suicide Risk Assessment Guide (SRAG) will be used as a teaching template for each of the sections of suicide risk assessment. Working through the SRAG will help you consolidate the information in the previous chapter in a clinically meaningful manner.

The Suicide Risk Assessment Guide (SRAG)

The SRAG is a four-page summary of the information contained in this section that can be used to guide the clinical interview for the evaluation of individual suicide risk. The SRAG is available in Appendix 1, and you may wish to photocopy it and have it available as you work through this section. This will help you to learn how to use the SRAG effectively and then you will be able to use it in your own continuing health education, in reviews of patients, and in specific learning situations such as team-based case reviews. At the conclusion of this section a summary tool called the Tool for the Assessment of Suicide Risk (TASR) will be described. This tool collapses the information found in the SRAG into a simple, time-efficient instrument that can be readily applied in clinical care settings.

For each section of the suicide risk assessment discussed below the corresponding component of the SRAG is illustrated and instruction for completion of the respective component is provided. Many of the sections contain a summary suicide risk assessment rating wheel. Each wheel is divided into quadrants by a vertical and horizontal axis. This rating wheel is constructed to help you weigh the balance of risk for each section of the assessment. The upper right quadrant is generally indicative of highest risk and the bottom left quadrant as lowest risk for the factors being evaluated.

Example

Psychiatric diagnosis and symptom suicide risk assessment guide (SRAG) rating wheel: symptoms/disorder evaluation

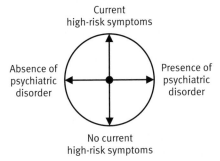

For a patient with a diagnosis of schizophrenia who presents with depressed mood and hopelessness:

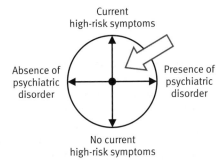

For a patient with depressed mood and hopelessness with no psychiatric diagnosis:

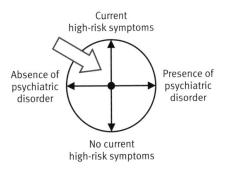

The suicide risk assessment

Any patient who expresses suicidal ideation must have a thorough suicide assessment to evaluate suicide risk. Unfortunately, some people who are contemplating suicide may be reluctant to reveal suicidal thoughts to their regular health-care provider even when asked directly. They may be even less likely to reveal suicidal thoughts to a clinician with whom they do not have a therapeutic relationship. Failure to disclose suicidality is a particularly pertinent issue for clinicians in casualty departments where they are often faced with having to assess suicidality in patients whom they are meeting for the first time.

Question

Who needs an assessment?

Answer

Although some of the risk factors discussed above may be of limited utility in identifying which patients will or will not commit suicide, these risk factors can be useful in identifying which patients must be assessed for suicidality. Individuals who have made a suicide attempt or engaged in other self-harm behaviours and those who express suicidal thoughts and/or hopelessness should be assessed as soon as possible. Patients who engage in self-destructive behaviours such as self-mutilation (cutting, burning) should also be assessed because such behaviours may be motivated by underlying suicidal thoughts or plans. Patients who are diagnosed with a serious physical illness should also be assessed, particularly if the illness is life threatening, may cause disfigurement, is associated with severe pain or loss of functioning, and is accompanied by psychiatric symptoms.

Any patient with a psychiatric illness should be evaluated for suicidality periodically throughout their illness course regardless of their clinical status. However, there are particular times in the patient's illness course that may be associated with higher suicide risk and call for a higher index of suspicion on the part of the health-care provider.

Question

For patients suffering from a mental disorder, when should an evaluation for suicidality be performed?

Answer

Suicidality **must** be evaluated...

- When patients present in crisis to mental health or casualty services.
- During all initial psychiatric inpatient or outpatient clinic evaluations.
- When a change in patient observation status or treatment setting is contemplated. For example, prior to discharging any patient from an inpatient unit, prior to changing patient hospital privileges (i.e., discontinuation of one-on-one observation or provision of patient passes outside of hospital), or discharging patients from the emergency room setting.
- When there is a sudden change in clinical presentation. Any patient who experiences a sudden decompensation or worsening in their symptoms must be assessed for suicide risk. Any patient who experiences a sudden unexpected improvement in symptoms must also be assessed for suicide risk. Some patients, particularly those suffering from depressive illness, may feel a sense of relief and joy after making the decision to end their life. Death may be a welcome escape from what is perceived and experienced as endless suffering and unremitting pain. To some, the decision to suicide may symbolize regaining of control over their lives and releasing the burden of their illness. To others, death may be seen as a way to reunite with lost loved ones, to reach utopia or experience a rebirth into a better life.
- When patients fail to experience improvement or experience a worsening of their symptoms despite treatment.
- When the patient has experienced an actual or perceived loss, has suffered shame or humiliation, or has been exposed to another significant psychosocial stressor. Attempts to understand the patient's experience from the patient's perspective is important. Subjective experiences of similar events are highly variable. For example, the death of a relative may be devastating to one individual but have minimal effect on another. Similarly, for some individuals anticipated or perceived loss may be as stressful as actual loss. For example, to some, the threat of loss of a relationship can be as overwhelming as the experience of actual termination of the relationship. Likewise, what is experienced as shame or humiliation and how shame and humiliation are addressed may be culturally bound. Understanding what an experience means to the individual, taking into account the patient's familial, cultural and societal context, can provide important insights for the evaluation of suicide risk.

Learning how to assess suicide risk

The goals of the assessment are to identify individual suicide risk and protective factors in order to estimate suicide risk (calculate the 'burden' of risk); to gain an appreciation of and help the individual gain insight into his or her motivation to suicide; to identify modifiable factors amenable to interventions; and to target interventions to reduce suicide risk.

Four steps in the assessment of suicide risk:

Step I   Assessment of suicidality
Step II Evaluation of suicide risk factors
Step III Identifying what's going on
Step IV Identifying targets for intervention

Summary of the four steps

Step I: Assessment of suicidality

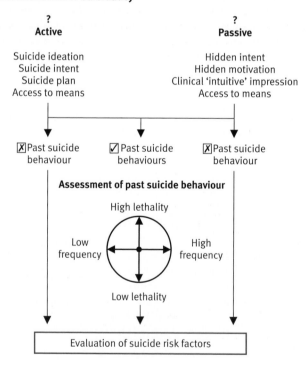

Step II: Evaluation of suicide risk factors
1 Patient information: age and gender.
2 Past and current suicidality.
3 Psychiatric diagnosis and psychiatric symptoms.
4 Individual history:
a medical history;
b family history;
c psychosocial history;
d neurobiology.
5 Personality strengths and weaknesses.

Step III: What's going on?
When conducting a suicide risk assessment, look for possible answers to the following questions:
• Why?
• Why now?
• What's going on?

Identifying answers to these questions will help the health professional to understand the complexities of factors underlying or precipitating suicidal behaviours. This in turn will facilitate the identification of targets for intervention.

For most patients the answers to these questions can be categorized as follows.

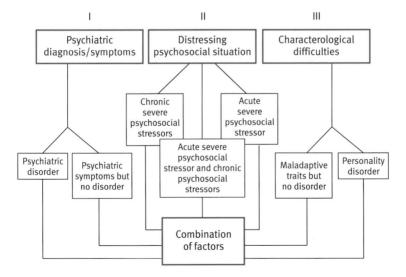

Step IV: Intervention
Identify and target interventions to reduce modifiable suicide risk factors.

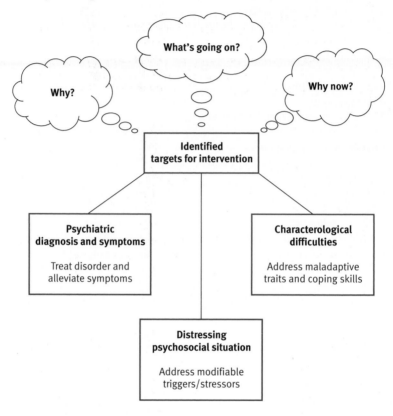

Step I: Assessment of suicidality

Initiating the suicide assessment
How to talk to patients in order to establish suicidality

Establishing rapport with the patient is the initial approach to any medical assessment but particularly one involving a patient who presents with suicidality (suicidal ideas, suicide plan or a suicidal attempt). Use of a calm, patient, non-judgemental and empathic approach will help create a safe and comfortable atmosphere for the patient.

As health professionals it is important to recognize that working with or assessing a suicidal patient, whether in a community office or in the accident and emergency department, can be influenced by a clinician's reactions to or feelings about the suicidal patient and/or about suicide in general. Clinicians may experience a variety of reactions when confronted with the suicidal patient including feelings of helplessness, anger, anxiety, disappointment, ambivalence, sadness, ineptitude or rejection. It is important that clinicians do not allow such feelings to influence their professional assessment and treatment of the patient.

Begin your assessment with empathic, nonthreatening statements and inquiries. This makes it easier for the person to share how they are feeling and thinking with you. Once the patient feels more comfortable in the interview situation they are more likely to disclose thoughts and plans about suicide to the clinician. The following are some examples.

The empathic statement

I can see how difficult things have been for you lately...
It seems that things have been hard for you and that it has been difficult to cope...
You seem to be having a hard time...

The gentle inquiry

I wonder if you would help me understand how this has been for you?
Can you share your concerns with me?
Can you tell me about what has been happening?
How have things been for you lately?

When beginning the assessment start with general questions about suicidal thoughts or wishes before focusing on more specific details. Because the patient may minimize the severity or even the existence of suicidal thoughts it could be necessary to take different approaches to questioning about suicidality or to revisit questions about suicidality at different times during the interview.

Once you have established rapport with the person, then you can go ahead to ask more specific questions about suicide. These should begin with questions to elicit suicidal ideation, then suicidal intent, followed by suicide plans.

What not to do

1 Avoid rushing the patient or asking leading questions such as:
   You don't have any ideas about suicide, do you?

Such questions convey an attitude of dismissal, judgement and disinterest on the part of the clinician. Even if the patient is acutely suicidal he or she is unlikely to feel safe enough in such a situation to disclose honest intention.

2 Do not 'interrogate' the patient or force the patient to 'defend his or her action':
Why would you do such a thing?
Why would you even consider suicide?
What is wrong with you?
What is so bad in your life?

3 Do not minimize the patient's distress:
Oh, you are fine.
It's not such a big thing is it?
Lots of people go through these kinds of things and are fine!

4 Do not undercut the seriousness of the suicidal thoughts or behaviour:
Come on… you are not really going to do anything.
If you really wanted to die you would be dead by now.
You'll feel better after a good night's rest.
Get over it… you are fine.

Do not avoid asking directly about suicidality even if you think the responses would be negative!

Bottom line

ASK THE QUESTION!!

Be sensitive and non-judgemental in your approach but don't avoid asking:
'…Have you ever thought about harming yourself?'
'…Have you ever tried to do anything to yourself that could have seriously harmed you or killed you?'
'… Have you been thinking about killing yourself?'

Remember:

If the person has been having thoughts about death, feelings of hopelessness, or committing suicide, addressing these issues openly in a calm, non-judgemental, empathic manner can be a great relief for that person. Creating an opportunity for open dialogue also creates opportunity for discovering new alternatives and choosing differently.

Acquiring collateral information

Patients may deny the presence or degree of suicidality in the clinical situation, particularly in the acute care setting or when dealing with clinicians they do not know. It is therefore essential that collateral information be obtained from individuals who are well acquainted with the patient. Family members, friends, health professionals, teachers, staff or clergy may be valuable resources for the clinician performing the assessment. These individuals can provide essential information that may influence the clinician's determination of patient risk. Remember that many people who die by suicide communicate their intent to others within six months of the attempt. Informants can provide important information about recent and past expressed suicidality as well as the patient's psychosocial history, current life circumstances, psychiatric and medical history, description of past self-injurious behaviours or suicide attempts, family environment and family history of suicide or mental illness, personality strengths and vulnerabilities, and ability to use coping strategies and mobilize external supports during times of stress.

Question

What if the person does not directly answer questions about suicidality and I think the person is at risk but there is no one available to provide reliable collateral information?

Answer

Some people who are suicidal will not openly disclose suicidal ideation, intent or plans. These patients may demonstrate 'passive suicidality'. In these situations collateral information is especially important as described above. If collateral information is not available the clinician must rely more heavily on clinical judgement based on apparent risks, possible 'warning signs' and subjective impression.

What to do

1 Look for 'warning signs' of possible hidden suicidal ideation, intent, or plan:
   - evidence of psychosis;
   - unable to develop rapport with the individual;
   - avoids eye contact during interview;
   - reluctant to answer direct questions about suicidality;
   - responds with 'I don't know' to questions about suicidality;
   - appears despondent or emotionally distant;
   - appears angry or agitated.

2 Look for evidence of past self-harm behaviours in the patient's hospital records (e.g. past suicide attempts and suspicious injuries that may have been unreported attempts) or during the physical exam (e.g. scars from self-inflicted lacerations).

3 Complete the suicide risk assessment even if much of the information is not available.

4 Place particular emphasis on the evaluation of current high-risk psychiatric symptoms and on uncovering the presence of a possible psychiatric disorder that may place the individual at high risk.

5 Err on the side of caution when making decisions regarding disposition and intervention... If your gut says something is not right, something is probably not right!

Assessment of current suicidality
Assessing suicidal ideation

Suicidal ideation refers to thoughts, fantasies, ruminations and preoccupations about death, self-harm and self-inflicted death. The greater the magnitude and persistence of the suicidal thoughts the higher the risk for eventual suicide.

In order to determine the nature and potential lethality of the patient's suicidal thoughts, it is necessary to elicit the intensity, frequency, depth, duration and persistence of the suicidal thoughts. Even if the patient initially denies thoughts of death or suicide, the clinician should ask additional questions if she or he feels the patient is not being forthcoming or is at high risk. Asking patients how they feel about the future or if they have been making or anticipating future plans may provide useful insights. Patients who are considering suicide may be ambivalent or fatalistic about the future, may describe a future devoid of hope, may express despair about the future or may not think about the future at all.

Remember that asking patients about suicidal thoughts does not plant or nurture these thoughts or wishes in the patient's mind. Rather, patients often feel relieved that they have finally been given 'permission' to talk about these thoughts and feelings. Many patients who have suicidal ideation feel burdened, ashamed and sinful for having such thoughts. Some are frightened by them. Some interpret these thoughts as reinforcements for their own perceived worthlessness. Opening the door to open dialogue about such thoughts and fears offers patients the opportunity to be heard and to feel understood, and can help to alleviate patients' psychological and emotional stress.

Asking about suicidal ideation

(Remember: start general then become more specific)

Do you ever feel that life is not worth living?
Do you ever have thoughts about not wanting to live anymore?
Do you ever wish you were dead?
Is death something that you have thought about recently?
Do you ever think about ending your life?

Assessing suicide intent and plan

Suicidal intent refers to the patient's expectation and commitment to die by suicide. The strength of the patient's intent to die may be reflected in the patient's subjective belief in the lethality of the chosen method, which may be more relevant than the chosen method's objective lethality.

The clinician must attempt to elicit the presence or absence of a suicide plan including when, where and how a patient intends to commit suicide. This information will help inform the clinician of the potential lethality of the plan and the possibility of its success. More detailed plans are generally associated with a greater suicide risk. The lethality of the chosen method, the patient's knowledge and skill regarding the method, the absence of intervening persons or protective circumstances, the patient's preparedness to carry out the plan, the patient's access to lethal means and the patient's commitment to die by suicide all must be considered when assessing suicidal intent/plan.

The patient's expectations and beliefs regarding the lethality of the chosen method for suicide are important to consider when estimating strength of intent. Even though the objective risk of a chosen method may be minimal, a patient's subjective conviction of the method's lethality places that patient at higher risk. The greater and clearer the suicidal intent the higher the risk for suicide.

Important aspects of a suicide plan that are suggestive of the plan's potential lethality include the following:

- Method
- Availability of means
- Patient's belief about the lethality of the method
- Chance of rescue
- Steps taken to enact plan
- Preparedness for death

Patients with higher degrees of suicidal intent, or more detailed and specific suicide plans, particularly those involving violent and irreversible methods, should be given a higher level of risk. If the patient has access to a firearm, or other lethal means, attempts should be made to ensure that these means are no longer available to the patient. Family members or other informants should be counselled to restrict access to, secure, or remove these means from the patient's environment.

Question

How do you ask about suicidal intent and suicide plans?

Answer

If someone has expressed suicide ideation, ask direct and specific questions about suicide intent and plans.

Have you felt that you or others would be better off if you were dead?

Do you feel that life is not worth living?

Do you wish that you were dead?

Have you had specific thoughts about how you might take your own life?

What have you thought about as a way to take your life? What other things have you considered?

Have you set a time, or date or place for taking your own life?

Have you obtained or do you have access to...

...pills?

...poison?

...medication?

...weapons?

Have you chosen...

...a place to hang yourself?

...a place to jump?

...another method that we have not discussed?

If you were alone right now, would you try to kill yourself? What about in the near future?

Assessing motivations for suicide

There may be multiple motivations for suicide for each individual patient. Delineating what these motivations are can help clinicians identify potential areas for intervention. Always ask 'Why?' and 'Why now?'

Common examples include the following:

- Anger toward others that is redirected toward self.
- A means to escape from suffering.
- A wish to be reunited with loved ones.
- Hopelessness.
- Recent loss of a relationship.
- Shame or humiliation.
- Manipulation.

Clinical application

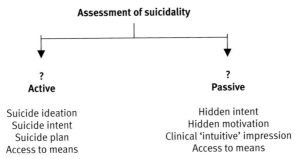

The SRAG: assessment of current suicidality

Rate current intensity, frequency and persistence of suicidal ideation as low (1), medium (2) or high (3) by placing a check in the corresponding column:

Assessment of current suicidal ideation

Current suicidal ideation	☐ Intensity	1	2	3
	☐ Frequency	1	2	3
	☐ Persistence	1	2	3

By placing a check in the corresponding column, rate each item listed as low (1), medium (2) or high (3).

Assessment of current suicidal intent and plan

Current suicide intent & plan	☐ Expectation & commitment to die	1	2	3
	☐ Lethality of method	1	2	3
	☐ Availability of means	1	2	3
	☐ Patient's belief in lethality of method	1	2	3
	☐ Chance of rescue	1	2	3
	☐ Steps taken to enact plan	1	2	3
	☐ Preparedness for death	1	2	3

By placing a check in the corresponding column, rate each item listed as low (1), medium (2) or high (3).

Assessment of past suicidality

Past suicidal behaviour, including history of suicide attempts, aborted attempts or other self-harming behaviour, is a significant risk factor for suicide. When assessing a patient who has a history of a previous suicide attempt or self-injurious behaviour it is important to obtain as much detail as possible about the number of past suicidal behaviours; the timing, intent, method and consequences of such behaviours; the life context in which they occurred; whether they occurred in association with intoxication or chronic use of alcohol or other substances; and the patient's current feelings about the behaviours.

Question

How do you assess past suicidal behaviours?

Answer

In evaluating past suicidal behaviours, the following information must be obtained:
- Type of past suicidal behaviours
- Frequency of past suicidal behaviours
- Lethality of past suicidal behaviours

Type of past suicidal behaviours

Remember that there are many suicidal variants, therefore inquiry into past suicidal behaviours must include questions about past attempts for which help was sought or that came to the attention of health professionals, past attempts that have remained hidden, failed attempts, aborted attempts (during which the patient changed his or her mind), manipulative gestures, and other self-harm and risk-taking behaviours.
- Previous detected suicide attempts.
- Previous undetected suicide attempts.
- Aborted suicide attempts.
- Self-harming behaviours.

Frequency of past suicidal behaviours

The more frequent the attempts the higher the risk for completed suicide, even if the lethality of the events has been low or moderate (e.g. wrist slashing, taking handful of benzodiazepines, etc.). In addition to inquiring about the number of past behaviours, it is important to note any changes in the frequency of behaviours.

Lethality of past suicidal behaviours

Understanding 'lethality' necessitates an appreciation of the nature and severity of past suicidal behaviours as well as the 'intent' of past behaviours. Remember that one severe past suicide attempt increases the risk of subsequent success.

Nature and severity

An appreciation of the nature and severity of past attempts can be gleaned from gaining an understanding of the 'context' in which the behaviours occurred, the lethality of methods chosen, and the consequences of past behaviours.

Context

Information to elicit from the patient or informant regarding the context of past suicidal behaviours:

1 Intoxication at time of events:
   Was the use of alcohol or another drug associated with the attempt?
2 Interpersonal circumstances:
   Was the episode the result of an impulsive act perhaps associated with an argument or some other affective storm?
3 Events leading up to the behaviours:
   Was there a specific trigger such as loss of a job, loss of a relationship, etc....?
4 Time and setting of past behaviours:
   Was the episode planned for some time with great attention taken to choice of location and method?
5 Impulsivity of past behaviours:
   Was the event driven by impulse or anger?
6 Planning of past behaviours:
   Was the event planned or detailed?
7 Chance of discovery:
   Did the patient choose a situation in which the chance of discovery was low?
8 Persons present at the time of the behaviour:
   Who if anyone else was present?
9 Persons to whom the attempt was communicated:
   Who if anyone knew about the plan before the event?
10 How the attempt was averted:
   Why did death not occur?
11 Affect following the event:
   Was the person relieved or disappointed that they did not die?

Method

Information to elicit from the patient or informant regarding the methods chosen during past suicidal behaviours:

1 Lethality of method:

Did the patient choose a highly lethal method, such as a gun, hanging, poison, gas, etc.? Jumping from a significant height, shooting oneself with a gun or taking an agricultural poison are all examples of very lethal means. On the other hand, cutting the wrist with a safety pin is an example of relatively nonlethal means.

2 Insight into lethality of method:

Did the patient know that the means chosen was very likely to lead to a deadly outcome (e.g., if the patient took a handful of iron supplements, did she know that ingestion of a bottle of iron tablets could be fatal)?

If a method of low lethality was chosen, did the patient believe he or she would die as a consequence of the chosen method (e.g., if the patient ingested a handful of nonlethal pills)?

Consequences

Information to elicit from the patient or informant regarding the consequences of past suicidal behaviours:

1 Medical severity

Did the event result in:

–medical intervention in the emergency department?

–admission to a medical ward?

–intensive care?

–ongoing physical health consequences?

2 Treatment consequences

Did the event result in:

–admission to an inpatient psychiatric ward?

–referral to outpatient mental health?

–prescription of psychiatric medication?

3 Psychosocial consequences

Did the event result in:

–job loss?

–loss of relationship?

–legal issues?

–other negative outcome?

Intent

This entails an evaluation of how serious the patient was about dying. In other words, was the suicide attempt really an attempt by the patient to take his or her life or was it a gesture of frustration or anger in which the patient did not really want to die?

The following information should be elicited from the patient or informant in order to determine the patient's intent to die:

1 Expectation of lethality of the chosen methods
  Did the patient believe the method to be lethal?
2 Ambivalence toward living
  Did the patient really want to die?
3 Feelings about past suicidal behaviour
  Feelings about discovery:
  –is the patient relieved that he or she was discovered?
  –was the patient disappointed that he or she was discovered?
  –did the patient's attempt and subsequent discovery strengthen his or her resolve to die in the future?
  Feelings about survival:
  –is the patient relieved that he or she did not die?
  –was the patient disappointed that he or she did not die?
  –did the patient's attempt and subsequent failure strengthen his or her resolve to die in the future?

Clinical application

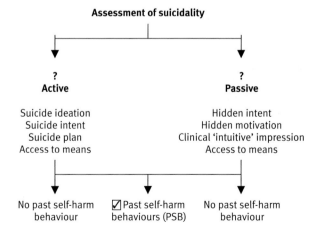

The SRAG: assessment of past self-harm behaviours
Past self-harm behaviours rating

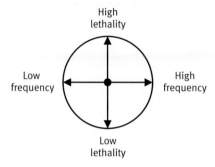

Assessment of past self-harm behaviours

	Suicide Motivation: *Why & Why Not?*		
High lethality / Low frequency / High frequency / Low lethality ⟱ **Past self-harm behaviours**			
		Number	Lethality
	☐ Past suicide attempts		1 2 3
	☐ Past self-harm behaviours		1 2 3

Check the boxes next to those items that apply to the individual; record the number of events in the next column, and then rate each checked item as low (1), medium (2) or high (3) lethality.

Step II: Evaluation of suicide risk factors

Psychiatric history and psychiatric symptoms
Psychiatric disorder is the single most attributable risk factor for suicide.

Establishing the patient's psychiatric history (i.e., previous psychiatric diagnoses and treatments, illness onset and course, and previous psychiatric hospitalizations), and conducting a careful psychiatric mental status examination to identify current psychiatric signs and symptoms is essential. As greater risk is associated with depressive, anxiety, substance abuse and psychotic disorders, particular attention should be placed on the evaluation of symptoms characterizing these syndromes.

Psychiatric symptoms
Psychiatric symptoms associated with greater risk of suicide:
- Severe anxiety
- Panic attacks
- Hopelessness
- Command hallucinations
- Impulsiveness
- Aggression

Other symptoms that may increase suicide risk:
- Depression/dysphoria
- Severe anhedonia
- Shame or humiliation
- Decreased self-esteem
- Violence toward others
- Agitation
- Akathisia
- Anger
- Severe insomnia

Hopelessness
Hopelessness, whether in the presence or absence of clinical depression, raises the risk of suicide. When performing a suicide assessment interview the presence, persistence and degree of hopelessness must be evaluated.

One of the most significant symptoms associated with increased suicide risk is the presence of hopelessness.

   Individuals who experience 'hopelessness' may feel trapped by problems that appear unsolvable, situations that appear unchangeable, or pain that appears inescapable. They are often unable to see beyond their suffering and cannot grasp the possibility of better days to come.

Question

How do you ask about hopelessness?

Answer

Have you been feeling as if things will not change, not get better?
Have you been feeling as if it is just not worth trying any longer?
Are you pessimistic about your future?
Have you been feeling without hope – hopeless?

Assessing hopelessness

Do you ever feel hopeless?

Do you ever feel that things will not or cannot
ever get better for you?

Are there times when you cannot see
beyond your suffering?

Are there times when you are unable
to see any future for yourself?

No   **Yes**

How do you feel
about the future?   When you feel this way
do you ever wish
your life would end?

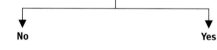

Where do you hope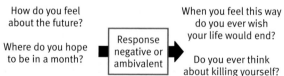
to be in a month?   Response
negative or   Do you ever think
ambivalent   about killing yourself?

What could you change
about your life right now
that would help you feel better?

Suicide risk assessment guide (SRAG) assessment of psychiatric symptoms and disorder

Clinical application
Assessment of suicide risk factors associated with psychiatric history and psychiatric symptoms (symptom risk factors section of the SRAG)

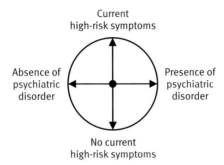

Current
high-risk symptoms

Absence of
psychiatric
disorder

Presence of
psychiatric
disorder

No current
high-risk symptoms

Assessment of suicide risk factors (SRF) associated with psychiatric symptoms

Symptom risk factors			
☐ Hopelessness	1	2	3
☐ Significant anxiety/panic attacks	1	2	3
☐ Command hallucinations	1	2	3
☐ Impulsivity	1	2	3
☐ Aggression	1	2	3
☐ Dysphoria	1	2	3
☐ Anhedonia	1	2	3
☐ Shame or humiliation	1	2	3
☐ Decreased self-esteem	1	2	3
☐ Agitation	1	2	3
☐ Akathisia	1	2	3
☐ Anger	1	2	3
☐ Severe insomnia	1	2	3

Place a check in the boxes next to those factors that apply to the individual then for each checked item rate the current significance to the patient from 1 to 3 where 1 = low significance; 2 = moderate significance; 3 = high significance.

Assessment of suicide risk factors (SRF) associated with ANY psychiatric disorder

Suicide risk factors (SRFs) for patients with ANY psychiatric disorder	Factor	1	2	3
	☐ Social isolation	1	2	3
	☐ Loss of family role/status	1	2	3
	☐ Interpersonal losses	1	2	3
	☐ Vocational/occupational loss	1	2	3
	☐ Loss of previous skills/competencies	1	2	3
	☐ Awareness of deficits with recovery	1	2	3
	☐ Substance or alcohol abuse/dependence	1	2	3
	☐ ↓ Problem solving capacity (cognitive impairment)	1	2	3
	☐ Depressive symptoms	1	2	3
	☐ Hopelessness	1	2	3

Place a check in the boxes next to those factors that apply to the individual then for each checked item rate the current significance to the patient from 1 to 3 where 1 = low significance; 2 = moderate significance; 3 = high significance.

Depression symptoms

☹ Depression symptom checklist	Symptom	1	2	3
	☐ Low mood	1	2	3
	☐ ↓ Interest in activities/↓ ability to feel pleasure	1	2	3
	☐ Significant change in weight	1	2	3
	☐ Sleep difficulties	1	2	3
	☐ Restless or slowed down	1	2	3
	☐ Fatigue/↓ energy	1	2	3
	☐ Feelings of worthlessness/guilt	1	2	3
	☐ Poor concentration or difficulty making decisions	1	2	3

Place a check in the boxes next to those symptoms that apply to the individual then for each checked item rate the current symptom severity from 1 to 3 where 1 = low; 2 = moderate; 3 = high.

Assessment of SRF associated with depression

Additional SRFs for patients with depression	Factor	1	2	3
	☐ Significant anxiety/panic attacks	1	2	3
	☐ Anhedonia	1	2	3
	☐ Psychosis	1	2	3
	☐ Return of energy early in recovery	1	2	3
	☐ Sudden clinical improvement	1	2	3

Place a check in the boxes next to those factors that apply to the individual then for each checked item rate the current significance to the patient from 1 to 3 where 1 = low significance; 2 = moderate significance; 3 = high significance.

Anxiety symptoms

Anxiety symptom checklist				
	☐ Excessive worry	1	2	3
	☐ Has difficulty controlling worry			
	☐ Restlessness	1	2	3
	☐ Fatigue	1	2	3
	☐ Poor concentration	1	2	3
	☐ Irritability	1	2	3
	☐ Muscle tension	1	2	3
	☐ Poor sleep (falling asleep/↑awakening at night)	1	2	3
	☐ Panic attacks	1	2	3

Place a check in the boxes next to those symptoms that apply to the individual then for each checked item rate the current symptom severity from 1 to 3 where 1 = low; 2 = moderate; 3 = high.

Assessment of SRF associated with anxiety

Additional SRFs for patients with anxiety				
	☐ Panic attacks	1	2	3

Assessment of SRF associated with schizophrenia

Additional SRFs for patients with schizophrenia				
	☐ Recent hospital discharge	1	2	3
	☐ Recovery following acute psychotic episode	1	2	3
	☐ Suicidal/violent command hallucinations	1	2	3
	☐ Akathisia	1	2	3
	☐ Agitation	1	2	3

Place a check in the boxes next to those factors that apply to the individual then for each checked item rate the current significance to the patient from 1 to 3 where 1 = low significance; 2 = moderate significance; 3 = high significance.

Substance use disorder symptoms

Current substance use: ☐ Alcohol ☐ Cannabis ☐ Other: _____

Substance use d/o symptom checklist:				
	☐ ↑ Problematic use	1	2	3
	☐ Use despite significant/recurrent consequences	1	2	3
	☐ Tolerance	1	2	3
	☐ Withdrawal	1	2	3
	☐ Past history abuse or dependence	1	2	3

Check or record type of substance use endorsed by individual. Place a check in the boxes next to those symptoms that apply to the individual then for each checked item rate the current symptom severity from 1–3 where 1 = low; 2 = moderate; 3 = high.

Assessment of SRF associated with substance use disorders

Additional SRFs for patients with any SUD		1	2	3
	☐ Recent, threatened or impending interpersonal loss	1	2	3
	☐ Presence of other psychiatric disorder	1	2	3
	☐ Presence of a depressive episode	1	2	3

Place a check in the boxes next to those factors that apply to the individual then for each checked item rate the current significance to the patient from 1 to 3 where 1 = low significance; 2 = moderate significance; 3 = high significance.

Assessment of SRF associated with alcohol use disorder

Additional SRFs for patients with alcohol use d/o		1	2	3
	☐ Continued or heavier drinking	1	2	3
	☐ Serious medical illness	1	2	3
	☐ Personality disturbance/psychiatric disorder	1	2	3
	☐ Other substance use	1	2	3

Place a check in the boxes next to those factors that apply to the individual then for each checked item rate the current significance to the patient from 1 to 3 where 1 = low significance; 2 = moderate significance; 3 = high significance.

Medical history

The medical history should focus on previous or current medical diagnoses and treatments. Obtaining a history of medical treatment can help identify medically serious suicide attempts as well as past or current medical diagnoses that may be associated with augmented suicide risk.

Characteristics of medical disorder associated with higher risk:

1 Chronic disease
2 Neurological disorder:
–associated with pain
–associated with functional impairment
–associated with cognitive impairment
–associated with loss of sight or hearing
–associated with disfigurement
–associated with increased dependence on others
3 Presence of a psychiatric disorder
4 Presence of psychiatric symptoms

Clinical application
Suicide Risk Assessment Guide (SRAG): assessment of associated medical disorders

Assessment of SRF associated with medical disorders

Risk factors for patients with medical disorders				
	☐ Chronic disease	1	2	3
	☐ Neurological disorder	1	2	3
	☐ Pain	1	2	3
	☐ Functional impairment	1	2	3
	☐ Cognitive impairment	1	2	3
	☐ Loss of sight or hearing	1	2	3
	☐ Disfigurement	1	2	3
	☐ Increased dependency on others	1	2	3
	☐ Presence of psychiatric disorder or symptoms	1	2	3

Place a check in the boxes next to those factors that apply to the individual then for each checked item rate the current significance to the patient from 1 to 3 where 1 = low significance; 2 = moderate significance; 3 = high significance.

Family history
Family history, particularly in first-degree relatives, of suicide or suicide attempts, or a family history of mental illness, including substance abuse, should be elicited. The circumstances of suicide or suicide attempts in the family should be discussed, including the patient's involvement and age at the time of suicide. A history of family conflict or separation, parental legal trouble, substance use, domestic violence, physical and/or sexual abuse may also increase suicide risk.

Question

How do you ask about a family history of suicide?

Answer

Because we know that suicide attempts and completed suicide 'run in families', it is very important to determine what suicide-related behaviours or events have occurred in the patient's family. In some cases the patient may not be aware of the information. In other cases the patient may be aware of the events that have occurred but may be reluctant to share the information for a variety of reasons including shame, fear of stigma or discrimination, and a need to protect the family.

Establishing rapport with the patient is essential. Use of a calm, patient, non-judgemental and empathic approach will help to create a safe and comfortable atmosphere for the patient and will facilitate disclosure.

Remember: Suicide is an extremely sensitive subject in any culture, and the myths, stigma, secrecy and shame surrounding suicide in families provide a powerful incentive to 'keep the secret hidden'.

Be gentle and reassure the patient that the information provided is confidential and that you are experienced and competent in dealing with such sensitive issues:

> Suicide-related behaviours in families are not uncommon... I have dealt with this issue with many individuals and families before, and it is OK to discuss this issue with me. Any information that we discuss here remains confidential.
>
> We know that some illnesses and even behaviours, like suicide, may run in families. In your wider family (parents, grandparents, aunts, uncles, brothers, sisters) has anyone ever committed suicide?
>
> Has anyone ever attempted suicide?
>
> Can you tell me what you know about that?
>
> How does that affect you personally?

Suicide Risk Assessment Guide (SRAG): family risk factors

Clinical application
Assessment of suicide risk factors (SRF) associated with family history

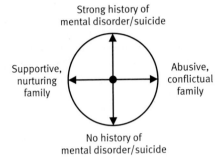

Assessment of SRF associated with family history

Family risk factors		1	2	3	
	☐ Suicide or suicide attempts in family	1	2	3	
Strong history mental d/o or suicide	☐ Suicide or suicide attempts in 1st degree relative	1	2	3	
	☐ Psychiatric disorder in family	1	2	3	
	☐ Psychiatric disorder in 1st degree relative	1	2	3	
Supportive ← → Abusive	☐ Substance use disorder in family	1	2	3	
	☐ Domestic violence/abuse	1	2	3	
Ø history mental d/o or suicide	☐ ↑ Family conflict	1	2	3	

Place a check in the boxes next to those factors that apply to the individual then for each checked item rate the current significance to the patient from 1 to 3 where 1 = low significance; 2 = moderate significance; 3 = high significance.

Psychosocial history
The goal of this component of the assessment is to gain an understanding of pertinent positive and negative psychosocial factors affecting the patient. Important aspects of the psychosocial history include delineation of the presence or absence of external supports available to the patient at home, at school, at work, at church or in the community; gaining an understanding of the patient's current living situation and what stressors or protective factors are currently present in that environment (e.g., whether there are young children at home; whether home is a pleasant

and comfortable place for the patient; the nature of the patient's current relationships with family, friends and colleagues; the presence of abuse or neglect); and gaining an understanding of the patient's employment status or school functioning. In addition, it is important to explore the patient's cultural and religious beliefs as they relate to death and suicide.

This component of the assessment also provides an opportunity for the clinician to identify both acute psychosocial crises and chronic psychosocial stressors currently affecting the patient. It is often useful to perform a quick screen of common psychosocial stressors as part of the assessment. Many patients are reluctant to disclose personal information about their lives spontaneously but may do so if specifically asked about particular areas of their lives.

Areas to explore with the patient include the following:
- Actual or perceived interpersonal losses
- Financial difficulties
- Changes in socioeconomic status
- Family discord
- Domestic violence
- Past or current sexual/physical/verbal/emotional abuse or neglect
- Housing problems
- Work problems
- School failure
- Perceived humiliation

Suicide Risk Assessment Guide (SRAG): assessment of psychosocial history

Clinical application
Assessment of suicide risk factors associated with psychosocial history

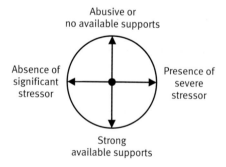

Assessment of SRF associated with psychosocial history

Psychosocial risk factors		1	2	3
☐ Actual/perceived interpersonal loss/bereavement		1	2	3
☐ Financial difficulties		1	2	3
☐ Changes in socio-economic status		1	2	3
☐ Family problems		1	2	3
☐ Marital/relationship problems		1	2	3
☐ Interpersonal/peer group problem		1	2	3
☐ Domestic violence		1	2	3
☐ Past or current abuse or neglect		1	2	3
☐ Housing problems		1	2	3
☐ Work/school problems		1	2	3
☐ Legal difficulties		1	2	3
☐ Perceived humiliation		1	2	3

Place a check in the boxes next to those factors that apply to the individual then for each checked item rate the current significance to the patient from 1 to 3 where 1 = low significance; 2 = moderate significance; 3 = high significance.

Personality strengths and vulnerabilities

It is important to gain an appreciation of the patient's strengths and vulnerabilities, ability to tolerate emotional or psychological stress, ability to utilize healthy coping strategies, individual personality traits and thinking style when estimating suicide risk.

Insight into potentially problematic personality traits or enduring patterns of behaviour may be identified by exploring reactions to past stressful life events (particularly past losses) with the patient or informant. Such an exploration may provide important information regarding the patient's ability to handle emotional and psychological stress, use healthy coping strategies, and mobilize internal and external supports

Areas to explore with patient and informant in the context of past stressors:

- Coping skills
- Personality traits
- Past responses to stress
- Capacity for reality testing
- Ability to tolerate psychological/emotional pain
- Ability to satisfy psychological/emotional needs

Suicide Risk Assessment Guide (SRAG): assessment of personality traits

Clinical application
Assessment of suicide risk factors associated with personality traits

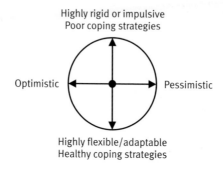

Highly rigid or impulsive
Poor coping strategies

Optimistic ← → Pessimistic

Highly flexible/adaptable
Healthy coping strategies

Assessment of SRF associated with personality traits

Personality risk factors		1	2	3
☐ History of poor coping skills		1	2	3
☐ History of poor problem solving		1	2	3
☐ Impulsivity		1	2	3
☐ Poor insight		1	2	3
☐ Poor affective control		1	2	3
☐ Rigid thinking		1	2	3
☐ Dependency		1	2	3
☐ Manipulative		1	2	3

(Personality risk factors diagram: Rigid/impulsive poor coping; Hopeful ← → Hopeless; Flexible/adaptive good coping)

Place a check in the boxes next to those factors that apply to the individual then for each checked item rate the current significance to the patient from 1 to 3 where 1 = low significance; 2 = moderate significance; 3 = high significance.

Suicide risk assessment summary

NAME: _____ Chart #: _____

INDIVIDUAL RISK PROFILE: ☆	YES	NO
Male		
Ages 15-35		
Age over 65		
Family history of suicide		
Chronic medical illness		
Psychiatric illness		
Poor social supports/social isolation		
Substance abuse		
Sexual/physical abuse		
SYMPTOM RISK PROFILE: ☆ ☆	**YES**	**NO**
Depressive symptoms		
Positive psychotic symptoms		
Hopelessness		
Worthlessness		
Anhedonia		
Anxiety/agitation		
Panic attacks		
Anger		
Impulsivity		
INTERVIEW RISK PROFILE: ☆ ☆ ☆	**YES**	**NO**
Recent substance use		
Suicidal ideation		
Suicidal intent		
Suicidal plan		
Access to lethal means		
Past suicide behaviour		
Current problems seem unsolvable to patient		
Suicidal/violent command hallucinations		

LEVEL OF SUICIDE RISK: High ☐   Moderate ☐   Low ☐

Assessment completed by: _____
(Name & position)
                                    DATE: _____

See Chapter 3 for instructions on completing this component of the SRAG, which is provided as a stand-alone summary tool called the Tool for Assessment of Suicide Risk (TASR).

Chapter 3

Putting It All Together: The Tool for Assessment of Suicide Risk (TASR)

Once you have completed Chapter 2 and understand the complexities of the suicide assessment, this section provides you with a short and succinct tool that summarizes the information contained in the SRAG in a format that can be used clinically when assessing a patient for suicidality.

The Tool for Assessment of Suicide Risk (TASR) (see Appendix 2) has been designed to be used by clinicians to document a summary of their assessment of a patient who may be suicidal. The TASR is divided into three sections: Individual Profile, Symptom Profile and Interview Profile; it may be used to ensure that the most pertinent individual, symptom and interview details necessary for the assessment of suicide risk have been addressed by the clinician. The TASR is thus a 'bedside' tool that helps the clinician determine the 'burden of risk' for suicide.

For each item listed check either 'yes' (applies to the patient) or 'no' (does not apply to the patient) in the corresponding columns to the right. Then rate the overall level of suicide risk as high, moderate or low by checking the corresponding box at the bottom of the table.

Note: The presence of a suicide plan or high suicide intent places the patient at high risk for suicide regardless of the presence or absence of any other risk factors.

The Tool for Assessment of Suicide Risk: TASR

NAME: _____ Chart #: _____

INDIVIDUAL RISK PROFILE: ☆	YES	NO
Male		
Ages 15-35		
Age over 65		
Family history of suicide		
Chronic medical illness		
Psychiatric illness		
Poor social supports/social isolation		
Substance abuse		
Sexual/physical abuse		

SYMPTOM RISK PROFILE: ☆ ☆	YES	NO
Depressive symptoms		
Positive psychotic symptoms		
Hopelessness		
Worthlessness		
Anhedonia		
Anxiety/agitation		
Panic attacks		
Anger		
Impulsivity		

INTERVIEW RISK PROFILE: ☆ ☆ ☆	YES	NO
Recent substance use		
Suicidal ideation		
Suicidal intent		
Suicidal plan		
Access to lethal means		
Past suicide behaviour		
Current problems seem unsolvable to patient		
Suicidal/violent command hallucinations		

LEVEL OF SUICIDE RISK: High ☐   Moderate ☐   Low ☐

Assessment completed by: _____
(Name & position)
                                    DATE: _____

© Dr. Stan Kutcher & Dr. Sonia Chehil, 2005

Guide to the Tool for Assessment of Suicide Risk

In the TASR, stars (☆) are used to provide the clinician with a section weighting of suicide risk. Section 1 is given a weighting of one star; section 2 a weighting of two stars and section 3 a weighting of three stars. The greater the number of stars, the greater the overall weighting of the section. The clinician should consider the weighting of each section as well as the scoring of items in each section.

Section I: Individual risk profile ☆

This section identifies age and demographic factors as well as pertinent family and personal medical and psychosocial history.

Many people have many of these risk factors but the majority of these individuals are not suicidal. These factors only have meaning when viewed within the context of the clinical presentation.

Factors within this section found to have the greatest correlation with suicide risk are listed in the box below.

> ## Individual risk profile
>
> Male
> Ages 15–35
> Age over 65
> Family history of suicide
> Chronic medical illness
> Psychiatric illness
> Poor social supports/isolation
> Substance abuse
> Sexual/physical abuse

Importance of this section in determining risk: ☆

Section II: Symptom profile ☆ ☆

This section addresses the **current** presence of psychiatric symptoms that have been associated with increased suicide risk.

Again, there are many individuals who experience some or many of these symptoms but the majority of these individuals are not suicidal. These symptoms must be viewed within the context of the clinical presentation.

Symptoms found to have the greatest correlation with suicide risk are listed in the box below.

Symptom risk profile

Depressive symptoms
Positive psychotic symptoms
Hopelessness or worthlessness
Anhedonia
Anxiety/agitation
Panic attacks
Anger
Impulsivity

Importance of this section in determining risk: ☆ ☆

Section III: Interview profile ☆ ☆ ☆

This section addresses acute factors identified during the interview that may place an individual at high risk of suicide whether accompanied or unaccompanied by other factors listed in sections I and II.

Risk is increased if risk factors from Section I are also present and risk is significantly increased if risk factors from Section II are also present.

Symptoms found to have the greatest correlation with suicide risk are listed in the box below.

Interview risk profile

Recent substance use
Suicidal ideation
Suicidal intent
Suicidal plan
Access to lethal means
Past suicide behaviour
Current problems seem unsolvable to patient
Command hallucinations

Importance of this section in determining risk: ☆ ☆ ☆

Section IV: Overall rating of risk

This section provides an overall rating of current individual suicide risk (the 'burden of risk'), which is rated as high, moderate or low based on the clinician's interpretation of information obtained.

LEVEL OF SUICIDE RISK: High ☐   Moderate ☐   Low ☐

Chapter 4
Suicide and Youth

Culture and society play an important role in determining what are considered normal trials and tribulations of adolescence in different settings. In many cultures, adolescence represents a time of change, of taking on new responsibilities, of planning and preparing for the future. It is also a time when many young people gain exposure to and experiment with 'different ways of being and expressing themselves'. Stressful life events and pressures from home, school, work, peers and community are all part of the normal process of growing and accumulating new experiences and life skills, and the vast majority of young people will negotiate their teen years and early adulthood successfully (some with a few hiccups along the way), and grow to lead fulfilling and productive lives. However, some young people have greater difficulty with the transition from childhood to adulthood. And some won't make it.

Suicide in young persons, like suicide in adults, is complex, with multiple dynamic interplaying factors contributing to the event in each individual case. Although the risk factor categories described in this monograph also apply to adolescents, there are risk factors that are particularly relevant to young people and deserve special consideration. These are addressed in this chapter.

In Western countries, suicide is often one of the top three causes of death in young people between the ages of 15 and 24. Risk for completed suicide is highest among older youth (late teens to early twenties), and in most countries boys are more likely to die by suicide than girls whereas girls make more suicide attempts than boys. In the USA, among 15–19-year-olds and among 20–24-year-olds the ratio of male to female suicide is estimated to be 4:1 and 6:1 respectively.

Depression is the strongest risk factor in teenage suicide.

The sharp rise in suicide rates in the adolescent years parallels the rise in the incidence of major mental disorders. It is estimated that up to 90% of young persons who suicide in the USA had a diagnosable mental disorder at the time of their death; for many, the disorder had been present for two or more years. Data from non-Western countries regarding this issue are generally unavailable and in subpopulations (such as aboriginal populations, and different ethnic, religious and cultural groups) these findings may not apply.

Psychiatric disorders most commonly associated with youth suicide include mood disorders (depression, hypomania-mania or mixed states), particularly when accompanied by alcohol or other substance abuse disorders, and disruptive behaviour disorders (particularly conduct disorder in boys). Depression is the strongest attributable risk factor in girls.

Psychiatric symptoms associated with higher risk of suicide in youth are similar to those in adults, with hopelessness, irritability, agitation, impulsivity and aggression being particularly significant. Other factors associated with higher risk include low self-esteem, poor self-confidence and a pattern of distorted negative self-appraisal and self-blame.

In addition to a history of suicidal behaviour and parental psychopathology (particularly depression and substance abuse), poor communication between the young person and his or her parents, rigid or unrealistic parental pressure or expectation, and rigid or unrealistic cultural pressure or expectation may also be important factors to consider when assessing suicide risk in teenagers.

Suicidal thoughts are relatively common amongst adolescents. Many young people will endorse contemplating 'ending their lives' particularly during or in the aftermath of a major stressor. Very few of these individuals will actually engage in deliberate acts of self-harm and even fewer will commit suicide. Suicidal ideation in and of itself does not indicate psychopathology or need for intervention in teenagers. In children, however, expression of suicidal ideation warrants serious attention. Young children may not appreciate the 'finality' of death and therefore may unwittingly commit suicide not realizing that they will not come back.

Suicidal behaviours, on the other hand, are more likely to be associated with psychopathology including mood and anxiety disorders, disruptive behaviour disorders and substance use disorders. Suicidal behaviours are more common in girls than in boys and are a significant risk factor for completed suicide in both sexes.

Suicidal behaviours are more common in girls than in boys.

Self-harm behaviours and completed suicide in adolescence is often preceded by a trigger (usually an acute psychosocial stressor) such as the breakup of a relationship, peer rejection, difficulties at home or trouble at school or with the law. In general, young people are more likely than adults to be short-sighted, impulsive and exhibit immature coping strategies particularly when under stress. It is always important to appreciate the significance of a stressor from the perspective of the individual, taking into account his or her sociocultural-religious background, experience, level of emotional maturity and psychological/cognitive sophistication. Stressors that may be of particular concern during adolescence include those associated with the following:

- Experience of or perceived shame or humiliation.
- Experience of or perceived bullying, social exclusion or rejection.
- Experience of or perceived failure.
- Experience of or perceived fear of loss of a loved one.

Question

There are many changes that take place during adolescence; how can you tell if the changes are benign or potentially dangerous?

Answer

In young people, differentiating between 'disturbance' that may be indicative of a major underlying problem and 'distress' that is relatively benign (a normal stress response to difficult life events and challenges) can be challenging even for the seasoned clinician. In hindsight, friends and relatives of young people who are found to be suffering from a mental disorder such as depression, substance abuse or schizophrenia will recall seeing 'warning signs' that something was not right in the months, or even years, before the individual accessed care and received a diagnosis. These 'warning signs' are often attributed to normal 'growing pains' until the underlying problem reaches a severity that necessitates help seeking.

Some of the 'warning signs' listed below are commonly expressed at one time or another by most, if not all, adolescents. Many of these warning signs are nonspecific and ambiguous, and taken separately may be just a normal part of growing up. On the other hand, if these warning signs represent a clear change in a young person's personality, behaviour or functioning they may be signals to a serious underlying problem. For example, changes in personality, behaviour or functioning may herald the onset of a neurological or psychiatric disorder (such as a seizure disorder, mood disorder, anxiety disorder, a substance use disorder, an undetected learning disability or more rarely schizophrenia); they may signal that the child or youth has or is experiencing a severe stressor or trauma; or they may be indicative of an underlying medical problem.

Warning signs that something may be wrong

- Significant changes in home, school, work or social function
- Significant changes in personality
- Significant changes in behaviour
- Withdrawal from family
- Withdrawal from friends and social activities
- Loss of interest in activities he or she once enjoyed
- Neglect of personal appearance
- Significant change in weight
- Sleep difficulties
- Persistent self-deprecating comments
- Use of drugs and/or alcohol
- Dysphoria, intense sadness or despair
- Increased irritability, anger or aggression
- Increased difficulty controlling emotion
- Increased risk-taking or impulsivity
- Preoccupation with death or people who have died by suicide
- Suicide or death as the theme of conversation, schoolwork or artwork
- Hopelessness as the theme of conversation, schoolwork or artwork
- Giving away valued possessions

How do you know when to be concerned?

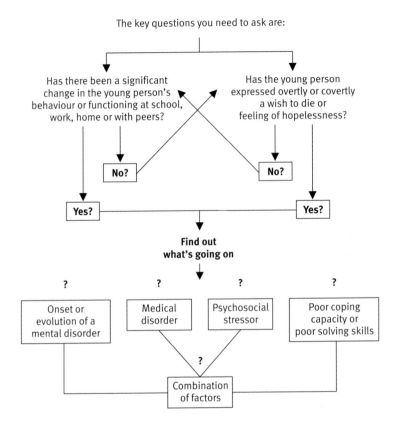

The key questions you need to ask are:

Has there been a significant change in the young person's behaviour or functioning at school, work, home or with peers?

Has the young person expressed overtly or covertly a wish to die or feeling of hopelessness?

No?

No?

Yes?

Yes?

Find out what's going on

?   ?   ?   ?

Onset or evolution of a mental disorder

Medical disorder

Psychosocial stressor

Poor coping capacity or poor solving skills

?

Combination of factors

As in adults, understanding these risk factors will not allow you to predict with certainty who will or will not commit suicide but it can assist clinicians in identifying young people who may be at risk for suicide, in performing a suicide risk assessment, and in determining the most appropriate level of intervention.

Family history of suicide and mental illness

As in adults, a family history of suicide or mental illness increases the risk for suicide in teenagers. Some youngsters may not be aware of this history, others may be very reluctant to share it. Obtaining this history from family members is essential. Always ask the teen and a family member (usually the mother if available) about a family history of suicide.

Collateral history and teen suicide

Many adolescents may be very reluctant to discuss suicidal ideation, intent or plans. This reluctance can be heightened in a situation in which the adolescent feels forced to comply or participate or when a teen does not relate to the health professional. Thus, a standard procedure when assessing a teenager should be to obtain a collateral history from a parent or other responsible adult (such as a teacher). However, a teenager should always be offered an interview separate from parents or guardians.

Confidentiality and the teenager

An adolescent may be reluctant to discuss personal information with a clinician particularly if the adolescent believes that he or she or their friends may 'get into trouble', or if the adolescent thinks that the clinician may tell their parents. Sometimes these fears may seem inconsequential to the clinician but will be very important to the teenager. For example, one teen whom S.K. interviewed was afraid his parents would find out that he had smoked a 'joint' at a party – a behaviour labeled as a 'sin' by his parents and the church to which he belonged. He had withheld discussion of his significant depressive symptoms and suicidal intent because of that issue, even though he had only once 'smoked a joint' and never used alcohol or other drugs. Confirmation of confidentiality allowed him to disclose his problems and he began treatment with good results.

As a clinical rule of thumb, it is useful to tell the teenager that information obtained in the interview will be held in confidence unless that information pertains to something that can seriously harm or injure the youth (such as suicidality). In such cases the responsible adult must be informed but the clinician must involve the adult in a manner that is respectful and protective of the young person.

Specific serotonin reuptake inhibitors (SSRIs) and adolescent suicide

An interest in the relationship between SSRI use and teenage suicide surfaced following a review of unpublished clinical trial data. Although some commentators (especially the media) struggled hard to forge a causal link between SSRI use and teen suicide, multiple independent investigations of the data by qualified groups and individuals showed that contrary to this perception, not only was SSRI use not associated with completed suicide but it was possibly a significant factor in treating teen depression and decreasing teen suicide.

SSRI use, however, can be associated with increased suicidal ideation and self-harm or suicidal behaviours in some teens. These medications should only be used by qualified health professionals with careful monitoring and proper patient/parent education.

The Kutcher Adolescent Depression Scale (KADS)

Many of the self-rated instruments often used to measure depression in adolescents (12–18 years) have limited or unknown reliability, validity and sensitivity to change over time in this age group. This is unfortunate because self-report scales have the potential to provide useful information quickly and cheaply. In view of the need for a quickly administered, valid, sensitive-to-change depression-rating scale for adolescents, one of the authors (S.K.) devised a self-report scale – the Kutcher Adolescent Depression Scale (KADS). The KADS is a validated tool that can identify teens who have depression and who may be suicidal. The original version of the KADS contained 16 items; the scale provided and described in this manual is the 6-item KADS.

The 6-item version of KADS was developed as a screening tool for depression in youth. This scale can be completed and hand scored quickly and easily and is ideal for screening and interview purposes in clinical settings.

The 6-item version of the KADS is reproduced in Appendix 3.

Assessing youth suicide risk: clinical summary

The following diagram provides a schematic overview of the clinical approach to mitigating teen suicide risk.

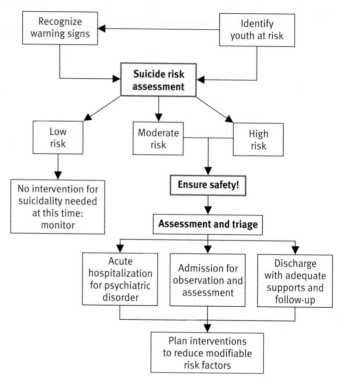

Clinical Assessment of Adolescent Depression (CAAD)

The Clinical Assessment of Adolescent Depression (CAAD) is a tool that was designed to accompany the 11-item version of the KADS. Once the youth has completed the KADS-11, clinicians can review and discuss the individual items of the KADS with the teen and an informant (usually a parent or guardian), if available, in order to gain a more comprehensive understanding of the teen's difficulties and to rule in or rule out a definitive diagnosis of depression.

In addition to reviewing the scores of the 11 items in the KADS completed by the teen (which are rated on a 4-point frequency scale from 'hardly ever' to 'all of the time'), clinicians are asked to have the teen and informant rate the severity of each symptom on a 4-point scale (0–4) where '0' represents the absence of the symptom; '1' is used to denote that the symptom is present but is experienced as mild and tolerable by the patient and is not associated with impairment; '2' is used to denote that the symptom is present, is moderate in severity, is experienced as problematic by the patient but does not significantly impair the patient's functioning; '3' is used to denote that the symptom is present and severe, difficult to tolerate and associated with significant impairment. Based on the information obtained from the teen and the informant the clinician also provides a 'composite' rating for each symptom using the same 4-point scale.

Additional items found in the CAAD that are not present in the KADS-11 include assessment of current substance use and an overall rating of symptoms, function and safety.

A copy of CAAD is reproduced and provided in the appendix.

Chapter 5
Commonly Encountered Problems in the Evaluation of Suicide Risk

The difficult patient

When dealing with suicidality, clinicians will come across two types of patients who can be particularly challenging to work with:
- The patient who presents repeatedly with low-lethality suicide attempts or self-harm behaviours.
- The patient who is chronically suicidal.

The frequent but low-lethality attempter and the chronically suicidal patient

Occasionally, clinicians will encounter a patient who exhibits frequent self-harm behaviours, often of low lethality, and who may have associated affective instability and/or deficient problem-solving skills. Such patients can be distressing to work with and clinicians charged with their care must learn how to appropriately assess, manage and treat such patients without allowing their own emotional responses to interfere with the quality of care provided.

Examples of 'low-lethality' self-harm behaviours include the following:
- Nonlethal cutting or burning of the skin, e.g., cuts or burns that are superficial or affect areas that do not endanger life.
- Nonlethal self-mutilation, e.g., cutting off an ear, digit, etc.
- Nonlethal overdosing on prescription or nonprescription medications, drugs or alcohol, e.g. ingesting five or six sleeping pills, taking three times the recommended dose of a prescription medication, ingesting a handful of vitamins.

When involved in the care of such patients remember:
- Past suicide attempts are a risk factor for suicide.
- Frequent low-lethality attempters do die by suicide.

- Many low-lethality attempters may have an underlying treatable mental disorder.
- Continued self-harm behaviours may be due to lack of response to ongoing interventions.
- Many low-lethality attempters may be in psycho-socio-cultural circumstances that are amenable to intervention.

Other patients may be 'chronically suicidal': that is, they may have daily thoughts of killing themselves. Although these patients may experience a waxing and waning of the intensity and persistence of these thoughts, periods of 'remission' of suicidality are often short-lived and strongly tied to psychosocial circumstances. These patients may or may not engage in self-harm behaviours.

When involved in the care of such patients remember:
- Suicidal ideation is a risk factor for suicide.
- It is a myth that 'People who talk about it don't actually do it'.
- People who are chronically suicidal do die by suicide.
- Many people with chronic suicidality may have an underlying treatable mental disorder.
- Chronic suicidal ideation may be due to lack of response to ongoing interventions.
- Many people with chronic suicidality may be in psycho-socio-cultural circumstances that are amenable to intervention.

These types of patients are challenging and will invoke ambivalent feelings in all clinicians at one time or another. As clinicians it is our responsibility to be aware of these feelings and not to allow these feelings to interfere with clinical care. The following guidelines may be helpful.

1 Be cognizant of your own emotional, cognitive and behavioural responses to these patients.
Common emotional responses:
- anger;
- hatred;
- frustration;
- disdain;
- helplessness;
- incompetence;
- anxiety;
- fear;
- resentment.

Common cognitive responses:
- *This person is weak.*
- *This person is disgusting.*
- *This person is a waste of time.*
- *This person is just trying to get attention.*
- *This person is taking advantage of me.*
- *This person is manipulating me.*
- *I wish this person would just die.*
- *I hate this person.*
- *I am incompetent because I cannot help this person.*
- *This person makes me feel useless and inadequate.*
- *If this person kills himself it will be my fault.*
- *I must protect this person.*
- *I must save this person.*

Common behavioural responses:
- avoidance;
- rejection;
- overinvolvement;
- overprotection;
- inappropriate assumption of a 'care-taking' or 'parental' role.

2 Learn how to manage your emotional and psychological responses so that you will be able to provide a thoughtful, non-judgemental assessment and make objective care decisions in the best interests of the patient. Obtain advice and consultation from an experienced colleague.

3 Avoid common traps.

Common traps:
- assumption of responsibility for the patient;
- creation of dependency;
- manipulation;
- exploitation;
- loss of personal boundaries;
- enmeshment (becoming overinvolved);
- enabling;
- burnout;
- avoidance.

Question

What can you do?

Answer

The first step is completion of a thoughtful, non-judgemental suicide risk assessment. This will allow you to make an informed evaluation of the patient's immediate risk for suicide. Focus on your cognitive, objective self, not your emotional, affective self.

For patients with limited or maladaptive problem-solving skills, suicidal behaviours may become an instrument used for interpersonal negotiations (sometimes referred to as manipulative suicidality) or a means of escape when faced with difficult problems whose solutions are not immediately apparent. Use of suicidality as an overt or covert threat in order to obtain attention, medication, admission, discharge, etc. from clinicians is not uncommon. Some of these patients may have a characterological disorder (such as borderline personality disorder) in which self-harm is a common part of the behavioural repertoire. Self-harm behaviours, such as nonlethal damage to the skin (e.g., burning or cutting) and nonlethal overdosing, are very distressing to families, friends and colleagues, who often have great difficulty in understanding and managing these behaviours and may become entangled in 'trying to keep the person safe' and thereby unwittingly become enablers of the very behaviour they wish to prevent.

It is important that patients, families and care-providers are able to differentiate between 'self-harm behaviour' and 'self-harm with the intention of suicide', keeping in mind that some individuals who 'self-harm' may purposely or by accident engage in self-harmful methods of fairly significant lethality (such as ingestion of large amounts of aspirin or acetaminophen), which may either result in death or cause significant physical damage without prompt medical intervention.

Psychiatric symptoms, such as hopelessness in depression or auditory hallucinations in psychosis, may underlie chronic suicidality. For patients not receiving treatment, initiation of appropriate treatment for the underlying symptoms by either psychotherapy (such as cognitive behaviour therapy for hopelessness) or medications (such as antipsychotics for schizophrenia) may ameliorate the suicidality. For patients receiving treatment a re-evaluation of current and past treatments, treatment efficacy, treatment compliance and treatment side effects is warranted, and lack of response or partial response to ongoing interventions should be addressed by optimizing or changing current treatment modalities. In some cases, 'hidden' psychiatric disorders such as bipolar type II or dysthymia may be present. Always consider this possibility in these individuals.

It is not uncommon for clinicians to find themselves manipulated and emotionally entangled with such cases, and many find it very difficult to maintain clinical perspective. Clinicians may inadvertently create dependency in the patient by falling into an ongoing care-giving or rescuing role. This type of relationship is unhealthy both for the clinician, who often becomes exhausted and resentful, as well as for the patient whose dependency is counter therapeutic.

> When feeling overwhelmed or having limited positive treatment effects – get a consultation from another clinician.

If past experience with the patient or the clinician's emotional responses to the patient are interfering with the objective assessment or management of the patient a request for a consultation should be made from another clinician. The results of the consultation should be openly discussed with the patient and others. Impressions regarding diagnosis and decisions on management and intervention must be unambiguous and clearly communicated to the patient, the patient's family and all members of the healthcare team, including those who may have intermittent contact with the patient in the community or the accident and emergency department, and documented in the patient's records.

Question

Why do individuals engage in self-harm behaviours?

Answer

The reasons are diverse and vary in each individual's case. Some patients describe feeling 'numb' or gaining a 'sense of relief' from psychological and emotional pain during and after self-inflicted physical pain or injury. Others report a brief feeling of euphoria associated with self-harm behaviours such as cutting. Some report using self-harm as a means of self-punishment, others as a means of decompressing anger. Some use self-harm behaviour as a means to control and manipulate others, particularly those with whom they are emotionally linked.

When a clinician is angry at a patient he or she may not be able to provide the careful, objective assessment of the suicide event that would otherwise be conducted. Thus, the first step in the assessment of these individuals is for the clinician to be aware of his or her own feelings about the case and to ensure as much as possible that these feelings do not get in the way of conducting an appropriate assessment of suicide risk. Remember, just because the patient has a long history of sublethal attempts does not mean that this time he or she is not serious. In all cases, a careful review and thoughtful non-judgemental exploration is necessary.

At the same time, care must be taken not to play into a manipulative scenario if that is present. The use of the lethality criteria noted above (in the TASR) is very valuable and will help guide clinical decision-making. If the clinician is not certain about the degree of the patient's risk then she or he may find it reasonable to provide for a short period of safe observation (ranging from a few hours to one day) during which the patient's risk for suicide will become more clear.

Chapter 6
Suicide Prevention

Suicide prevention strategies

There are essentially two types of strategies for suicide prevention:
* Population strategies
* Individual strategies

Population issues pertaining to suicide prevention

The most effective method for the prevention of suicide is the early identification and effective treatment by health-care providers of mental disorders, particularly mood disorders and alcohol- and other substance-related disorders, and secondly, the restriction of community access to highly lethal means. Depending on the population, this may entail such measures as detoxification of domestic gas; restricting access to firearms (particularly handguns); and reducing availability of toxic pesticides and herbicides (such as paraquat).

A number of interventions popularly considered as being very effective in reducing suicide rates, including suicide telephone hotlines and school-based suicide education programmes, have shown little or no substantial positive effect. The table below outlines the usefulness of a number of suicide intervention programmes for youth. The effect of national suicide prevention programmes when treatment (for depression and alcohol use) variables are controlled for is not clear. Improving the availability of mental health care may positively influence suicide rates.

Individual issues in suicide prevention

For the individual, suicide prevention methods should include early identification and appropriate treatment of mental disorders, recognition of warning signs of suicide risk, early identification and assessment of persons at risk for suicide, appropriate acute safety management for suicidal patients, and the implementation of targeted interventions for modifiable risk factors.

Usefulness of suicide intervention programmes for youth

No demonstrated benefit	Possibly harmful	Harmful	Likely benefit	Definite benefit
Suicide hotlines	School suicide awareness programmes	Sensational media coverage of suicides	School mental health awareness programmes	Early identification and treatment of mental disorders
School-based peer counselling programs	Focus groups or special school lectures on suicide		Restricted access to firearms and other available lethal means	Early identification and effective treatment of young people with suicide risk factors and warning signs
	Suicide screening in schools		Increasing and enforcing legal drinking age	Timely suicide risk assessment and focused intervention by health professionals

Chapter 7
Suicide Intervention

All patients identified as having warning signs or being at risk for suicide must have a comprehensive suicide assessment performed. Use of the Tool for the Assessment of Suicide Risk (TASR), which is described earlier in this manual, can assist clinicians in determining suicide risk, required level of care, and priority areas for immediate and ongoing intervention.

Basic principles underlying management of the suicidal patient

There are three basic principles to consider in managing the suicidal patient:
• Safety and security
• Support
• Targeted intervention

Safety and security

The first duty is to protect the patient from harm. For the acutely suicidal patient, admission to hospital or other similar facility may be necessary. For patients deemed high risk, involuntary commitment to a secure facility through legal means may be necessary if the patient is incompetent or if he or she refuses voluntary admission. All clinicians must be aware of the legal requirements regarding involuntary commitment in the jurisdiction in which they practice.

For the patient who has made an unsuccessful suicide attempt, medical assessment and stabilization using the basic principles of emergency intervention (A – airway, B – breathing, C – circulation) are priority actions. Treatment of identified medical issues such as electrolyte imbalances, heart irregularities, surgical intervention, suturing of lacerations, forced emesis in the case of medication overdose, etc. must be instituted. In many of these cases, hospitalization will be required.

If an acutely suicidal patient is hospitalized, the physician must ensure that hospital staff are fully aware of the patient's suicide risk and that the necessary precautions are taken to ensure patient safety. For example, the patient should not have access to means of self-harm (such as a belt that can be used for hanging, scissors that can be used for cutting, freedom of movement that can lead to jumping from a height). Patients who are highly suicidal may require constant or frequent observation and monitoring by responsible staff. The patient's level of suicide risk should be reviewed at least daily and decisions regarding freedom of movement and activity level (access to the general ward, interaction with other patients, participation in ward activities, off-unit privileges) should be made on the basis of this suicide risk review. A psychiatric or mental health consultation should be sought.

Question

What if a proper suicide assessment cannot be performed?

Answer

If a clinician is unable to complete an assessment or if he or she feels unsure of the patient's safety following completion of the assessment (even if the patient adamantly denies suicide risk) it is reasonable to admit the patient to a care facility and reassess in 8 to 12 hours. Suicidal patients who are intoxicated and are therefore unable to cooperate with an assessment should be held for observation until they have detoxified and a proper mental status examination can be carried out. In no case should a suicidal intoxicated patient be allowed to leave the clinic or hospital alone or in the company of anyone else.

Support

Patients with suicidal ideation or suicidal behaviours who do not require hospital admission should not be discharged unless appropriate arrangements for safety and supports can be put in place. In many cases, this will necessitate the cooperation of family or significant others. In such cases, patient safety takes precedence over patient confidentiality.

Family members, friends and significant others are usually very concerned about the patient's wellbeing and very distressed regarding the patient's behaviour. They are often unsure of how to behave, what to do or not to do, what to say or not to say, and how to help. Unless otherwise contraindicated, people who are close to the patient should be provided with psychoeducation about suicide and should be involved in decisions about hospitalization and in recommendations for immediate and long-term treatment.

If the clinician sends a patient with suicidal thoughts out of the hospital or clinic in the care of a responsible adult, care must be taken to ensure that the individuals to whom this responsibility of oversight is entrusted are capable of providing a safe, supportive environment and that they are informed of what to do if the patient's condition deteriorates. Care-givers should be advised to remove potential risks from the patient's environment. This may entail making medications, weapons or other lethal means inaccessible to the patient. It is advised that the patient and care-giver be instructed to return to the hospital immediately if there is an increase in suicidality.

In addition, the clinician should ensure that specific arrangements for reassessment and follow-up within 12 to 24 hours of discharge are made for the patient before the patient leaves the clinic or hospital and that safety precautions are available and in place in the interim. If a specialized psychiatric service is available, referral of the suicidal patient to this service is advisable. Whatever the arrangements, the clinician must always make a detailed note in the patient's chart explaining his or her action.

Question

What about the suicide prevention contract?

Answer

The suicide prevention contract may be used by clinicians in emergency rooms as well as acute and long-term inpatient and community settings. The success of the suicide prevention contract (sometimes referred to as the 'no harm' contract) is probably attributable to the strength of the therapeutic relationship between the patient and the clinician with whom the contract is formed. By itself, the 'no harm' contract has not been shown to be an effective preventive measure. In fact, it may give clinicians a false sense of security that may impair their ability objectively to assess suicide risk and may affect their judgement in terms of formulating treatment plans. The 'no-harm' contract is not a substitute for a proper clinical assessment and is not recommended for use in any clinical setting in which the clinician is faced with making clinical decisions about suicide risk with a patient with whom they do not have a strong therapeutic relationship. This is particularly important in the emergency and acute care setting. Suicide prevention/'No harm' contracts are also not recommended for use with agitated, psychotic, impulsive, intoxicated or cognitively impaired patients. When all is said and done, the assessment and treatment of suicidality relies on informed clinical judgement.

Targeted interventions

Once the assessment and the immediate safety management concerns are addressed, there are three areas of intervention that may be identified:

1 Serious mental disorders.
2 Acute and/or chronic psychosocial stressors.
3 Enduring maladaptive patterns of thought, emotion and behaviour.

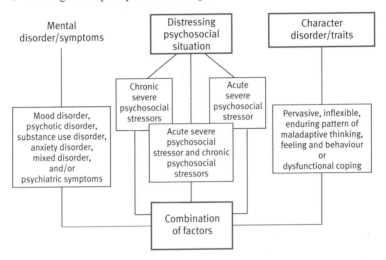

Many suicidal patients are found to have a treatable psychiatric illness. Appropriate treatment of an existing psychiatric disorder can significantly reduce suicide risk. In depression, for example, data from many studies clearly indicate that appropriate treatment with antidepressants, particularly the newer and safer SSRIs, decreases suicide rates. In psychotic patients with frequent suicidal behaviours treatment with the atypical antipsychotic clozapine has been shown to reduce suicide risk.

If a patient is found to have an untreated psychiatric disorder appropriate treatment should be initiated. For patients already receiving treatment for a diagnosed psychiatric condition treatment should be optimized following review of past and current treatment, treatment responses, treatment compliance and treatment side effects.

For patients whose suicidality is clearly linked to or exacerbated by severe psychosocial stress, provision of therapeutic support and/or temporary respite can allow the individual time and space to recover coping strategies, gain perspective and see options beyond suicide.

For patients with inadequate or maladaptive coping strategies, psychotherapeutic interventions that focus on skill building and problem-solving, such as cognitive behavioural therapy interventions, can be very helpful.

There is no 'cookbook recipe' that can be followed to treat the suicidal patient. It is the application of the above basic principles to the individual case that matters. In each case the clinician must determine the relative risk of suicide. The use of the TASR in this risk assessment can help the clinician in her/his task.

The cases found later in this manual (see Chapter 9) allow for the clinician, individually or as part of a self-study group, to practice application of the TASR and SRAG. The authors recommend that, following a reading of this monograph, the clinician immediately practice the application of the TASR or SRAG to at least two or three different cases so as to enhance learning of this material by its application.

Chapter 8
Post-suicide Interventions

Sometimes, in spite of our best interventions and the best possible care, an individual will commit suicide. The role of the care-provider does not end there. Don't forget that suicide does not occur in a vacuum. Once the individual ends his or her life, there are clinicians, family members, friends and communities that may require support.

Four principles of post-suicide interventions

The interventions that follow the suicide of an individual are based on four principles:

1 Support
2 Learn
3 Counsel
4 Educate

Support

This applies to the support that peers can give to their colleagues who have had the experience of one of their patients committing suicide. Such support need not be overbearing; a quiet recognition of the situation and availability to discuss how they are feeling is usually all that is required. Administrators or senior clinicians must make a concerted effort to provide this support to any health-care worker who reports to them. Often clinicians may blame themselves for the event or be shocked by it. Some people may respond by wanting to stop seeing patients. Others may become despondent. Gentle support will be much appreciated and very helpful.

Learn

It is always important to learn from the death of any patient, whatever the cause. Many hospitals have 'mortality rounds' in which objective review of fatal cases occurs as a learning exercise. In the case of suicide, such a learning review is also useful. It should be conducted in a supportive and non-judgemental manner and should follow prescribed procedures. Ideally this procedure should be described in the appropriate policies and procedures documents that guide services. Such sessions should involve groups of clinicians and be chaired by a senior clinician. Recommendations arising from such reviews should be taken into consideration for policy or service directions. The SRAG may be a useful tool to be used in such a review.

Counsel

In many cases the person who has suicided leaves behind a family or significant others. In such cases it is important to provide support and counselling to these individuals. Many may feel guilty or personally responsible. Some may be angry at the person who suicided. Whatever the affect or thoughts, offering a short period of supportive counselling (one or two meetings) in which individuals are able to discuss the event and mourn their loss is useful. These sessions can also help individuals to focus on practical issues that arise as a consequence of the suicide. For example, if a young child has been left by the suicide of a mother, what are the plans being put into place for proper care? Surviving children may need particular attention, and it is not unusual for them to experience a number of distressing symptoms such as bad dreams, sleep difficulties, somatic distress, etc. For some children, a longer period of support and counselling may be needed. These services can be provided by mental health professionals but they may also be provided or augmented by religious or community leaders. In that case, the mental health staff should communicate with those providing support and offer assistance in the form of training in useful therapeutic strategies if need be.

Educate

In some cases, such as the suicide of a prominent individual, the public interest in the event may provide an opportunity to educate others about suicide and the importance of identifying and treating mental illness. This can be an opportunity to address some of the issues around stigma – not only for suicide but also for mental illness in general. Particular attention should be paid to how this is done, especially if the media are involved. At no time should the health professional break patient confidentiality. Media interviews should use the event to focus on general issues and help both public and professionals understand rather than sensationalize. It is best if one senior person is identified as the media spokesperson. In situations where such an event happens in an institution (such as a school) there is no need for critical incident stress debriefing (it may do harm and there is no substantive evidence of it doing good). Instead support through group or individual interventions may be offered to students who require assistance. Usually, one or two meetings is all that is needed and the focus needs to be on the grieving process and not on other issues.

Health professionals should not use the media to promote their own personal beliefs or ideologies when addressing issues of suicide.

Chapter 9

Clinical Vignettes for Group or Individual Study

Cases: suicide assessment

The cases in this chapter have been developed to provide the reader with an opportunity to practice their suicide risk assessment skills. They are meant to be used as course material or continuing health education. They are best used in a group learning format. For each case, apply the Tool for Assessment of Suicide Risk (TASR) and come to a conclusion as to the level of risk: high, moderate or low. Then discuss your evaluation with your supervisor, teacher or fellow clinicians. Please also address issues of intervention – what you will do in each case – during the discussion. Remember to apply the TASR within the *context* of the case and using the ☆ weighting system.

Case One

Mrs J.S. is a 35-year-old housewife with a 19-year history of depression. This is her third episode. In previous episodes she improved with antidepressant medications usually within 4 to 6 weeks after beginning treatment. She has had no previous suicide attempts but her mother died of suicide many years ago. She is currently in a major depressive episode of some 2 months' duration and feels hopeless and worthless. She does not see any future for her children or herself and thinks that she would be better off dead. She is divorced and lives alone with her two sons who are aged 8 and 6 years. She has been taking an antidepressant medication for about two weeks and her mood is subjectively no better but she has more energy. Her major complaint (the reason why she came to see you) is painful headaches and she wants 'lots of strong painkillers'. At her last visit a week ago she told you she 'did not want to live with the black dog of depression any more'. Today she admits to feeling that 'life often does not seem worth living' and tells you that she has thoughts about killing herself. When you directly question her about suicidal plans she is vague and evasive in her response. When you ask how her children are doing she tells you that she has sent them to visit her ex-husband.

The Tool for Assessment of Suicide Risk: TASR

NAME: _____ Chart #: _____

INDIVIDUAL RISK PROFILE: ☆	YES	NO
Male		
Ages 15-35		
Age over 65		
Family history of suicide		
Chronic medical illness		
Psychiatric illness		
Poor social supports/social isolation		
Substance abuse		
Sexual/physical abuse		

SYMPTOM RISK PROFILE: ☆ ☆	YES	NO
Depressive symptoms		
Positive psychotic symptoms		
Hopelessness		
Worthlessness		
Anhedonia		
Anxiety/agitation		
Panic attacks		
Anger		
Impulsivity		

INTERVIEW RISK PROFILE: ☆ ☆ ☆	YES	NO
Recent substance use		
Suicidal ideation		
Suicidal intent		
Suicidal plan		
Access to lethal means		
Past suicide behaviour		
Current problems seem unsolvable to patient		
Suicidal/violent command hallucinations		

LEVEL OF SUICIDE RISK: High ☐   Moderate ☐   Low ☐

Assessment completed by: _____
(Name & position)
                                    DATE: _____

© Dr. Stan Kutcher & Dr. Sonia Chehil, 2005

Case Two

Mr M.I. is a 48-year-old unemployed male. About five weeks ago he had a heart attack from which he seems to have made a good recovery. He was discharged from the hospital about three weeks ago and has been at home since, mostly watching television and reading. He has come to see you complaining about back pain and constipation. At times during your interview he seems on the point of crying and he told you that he was very unhappy with how things are turning out for him. He says that his friends tell him it is common to be depressed after a heart attack. He tells you that his biggest interest right now is the church, in which he has been a member for over 20 years and talks about how his faith is very important to him and is sustaining him at this point in his life. He tells you that he is worried that he is losing his faith and talks about frequent anxiety attacks. On direct questioning he admits to having frequent thoughts about killing himself by taking all his heart pills at once but is worried that he will go to hell if he does. Yesterday he took a gun from its drawer and sat looking at it for about 15 minutes trying to decide if he should kill himself. He decided that his faith would not let him do it and that his wife would suffer if he committed suicide so he put the gun away.

The Tool for Assessment of Suicide Risk: TASR

NAME: _____   Chart #: _____

INDIVIDUAL RISK PROFILE: ☆	YES	NO
Male		
Ages 15-35		
Age over 65		
Family history of suicide		
Chronic medical illness		
Psychiatric illness		
Poor social supports/social isolation		
Substance abuse		
Sexual/physical abuse		
SYMPTOM RISK PROFILE: ☆ ☆	**YES**	**NO**
Depressive symptoms		
Positive psychotic symptoms		
Hopelessness		
Worthlessness		
Anhedonia		
Anxiety/agitation		
Panic attacks		
Anger		
Impulsivity		
INTERVIEW RISK PROFILE: ☆ ☆ ☆	**YES**	**NO**
Recent substance use		
Suicidal ideation		
Suicidal intent		
Suicidal plan		
Access to lethal means		
Past suicide behaviour		
Current problems seem unsolvable to patient		
Suicidal/violent command hallucinations		

LEVEL OF SUICIDE RISK: High ☐   Moderate ☐   Low ☐

Assessment completed by: _____
(Name & position)
                                    DATE: _____

© Dr. Stan Kutcher & Dr. Sonia Chehil, 2005

Case Three

Mr T. is a 46-year-old unemployed male with a known history of alcohol abuse and depression. He had his last depressive episode about 2 years ago and he was lost to follow-up after successful treatment with an antidepressant. He has not seen any health professional for at least one year and presents today to the emergency room complaining of abdominal pain. A physical examination is unremarkable and an X-ray of the abdomen shows no pathological findings. He lives alone and denies using any alcohol or drugs in the last month. His main concerns are about his physical health and he presents a variety of vague complaints about headaches and back pain after he is told that there is nothing to find regarding his abdominal pain. He denies being depressed but becomes tearful when talking about going back to the street where he has been living. He asks for food and the emergency room nurse complains that he is abusing the system.

The Tool for Assessment of Suicide Risk: TASR

NAME: _____ Chart #: _____

INDIVIDUAL RISK PROFILE: ☆	YES	NO
Male		
Ages 15-35		
Age over 65		
Family history of suicide		
Chronic medical illness		
Psychiatric illness		
Poor social supports/social isolation		
Substance abuse		
Sexual/physical abuse		

SYMPTOM RISK PROFILE: ☆ ☆	YES	NO
Depressive symptoms		
Positive psychotic symptoms		
Hopelessness		
Worthlessness		
Anhedonia		
Anxiety/agitation		
Panic attacks		
Anger		
Impulsivity		

INTERVIEW RISK PROFILE: ☆ ☆ ☆	YES	NO
Recent substance use		
Suicidal ideation		
Suicidal intent		
Suicidal plan		
Access to lethal means		
Past suicide behaviour		
Current problems seem unsolvable to patient		
Suicidal/violent command hallucinations		

LEVEL OF SUICIDE RISK: High ☐   Moderate ☐   Low ☐

Assessment completed by: _____
(Name & position)

DATE: _____

© Dr. Stan Kutcher & Dr. Sonia Chehil, 2005

Case Four

Mrs C. is a 23-year-old single actress who has not been able to obtain steady work in her profession since she moved to this city some 6 months ago. She supports herself by waiting on tables in a local bar. She has cut her wrists with a kitchen knife after an argument with the bartender with whom she has been living for the last 2 weeks. This is the third episode of wrist cutting she has experienced in the last 3 months. She also has cigarette burn marks on her upper arms and back and her face shows old bruises where she fell and hit her head while working. She does not have a history of depression or any other psychiatric disorder and before the above-mentioned episodes no history of self-harm behaviours. She does not drink or use drugs and is uncomfortable at her apartment because her boyfriend 'drinks too much' and 'gets loud'. She complains about feeling sad but denies being hopeless. She says she did not want to kill herself but cut herself because she did not know what else she should do.

The Tool for Assessment of Suicide Risk: TASR

NAME: _____ Chart #: _____

INDIVIDUAL RISK PROFILE: ☆	YES	NO
Male		
Ages 15-35		
Age over 65		
Family history of suicide		
Chronic medical illness		
Psychiatric illness		
Poor social supports/social isolation		
Substance abuse		
Sexual/physical abuse		

SYMPTOM RISK PROFILE: ☆ ☆	YES	NO
Depressive symptoms		
Positive psychotic symptoms		
Hopelessness		
Worthlessness		
Anhedonia		
Anxiety/agitation		
Panic attacks		
Anger		
Impulsivity		

INTERVIEW RISK PROFILE: ☆ ☆ ☆	YES	NO
Recent substance use		
Suicidal ideation		
Suicidal intent		
Suicidal plan		
Access to lethal means		
Past suicide behaviour		
Current problems seem unsolvable to patient		
Suicidal/violent command hallucinations		

LEVEL OF SUICIDE RISK: High ☐   Moderate ☐   Low ☐

Assessment completed by: _____
(Name & position)
DATE: _____

Case Five

Mr M. is a 19-year-old male who has taken a handful of aspirin tablets after an argument with his mother. This is his fifth episode of self-harm (always taking 'pills') in three years. He has never had a psychiatric diagnosis and in all previous cases he refused to see a psychiatrist or failed to show up for appointments after being seen in the emergency room. He has been in trouble with the law for selling drugs and for stealing from stores. His mother is a well-known political figure and she tells you that he is always trying to manipulate her into doing what he wants and always trying to 'get attention'. He denies any depressive symptoms but demands that you tell his mother to let him transfer to a new school because at his current school 'all the teachers are assholes'. He threatens to take more pills when he gets home if he is denied his demand.

The Tool for Assessment of Suicide Risk: TASR

NAME: _____ Chart #: _____

INDIVIDUAL RISK PROFILE: ☆	YES	NO
Male		
Ages 15-35		
Age over 65		
Family history of suicide		
Chronic medical illness		
Psychiatric illness		
Poor social supports/social isolation		
Substance abuse		
Sexual/physical abuse		

SYMPTOM RISK PROFILE: ☆ ☆	YES	NO
Depressive symptoms		
Positive psychotic symptoms		
Hopelessness		
Worthlessness		
Anhedonia		
Anxiety/agitation		
Panic attacks		
Anger		
Impulsivity		

INTERVIEW RISK PROFILE: ☆ ☆ ☆	YES	NO
Recent substance use		
Suicidal ideation		
Suicidal intent		
Suicidal plan		
Access to lethal means		
Past suicide behaviour		
Current problems seem unsolvable to patient		
Suicidal/violent command hallucinations		

LEVEL OF SUICIDE RISK: High ☐   Moderate ☐   Low ☐

Assessment completed by: _____
(Name & position)
                                        DATE: _____

© Dr. Stan Kutcher & Dr. Sonia Chehil, 2005

Case Six

Mrs P. is a 68-year-old woman with a five-year history of treated breast cancer. She lives with her 70-year-old husband who is very supportive of her. Her eldest daughter, her son-in-law and her two grandchildren live next door. She is very close to them all and visits daily. She has just been diagnosed with a recurrence of her cancer and broke down in her doctor's office, crying and saying that she does not want to live any more. She had a brief period of 'the blues' after her third child was born but has never been treated for any psychiatric problem. There is a strong history of depression in her biological family but no history of suicide. She denies having any suicidal plans and tells you that her thoughts about not wanting to live are gone. Now she feels embarrassed about having them and feels very upset. She denies feeling hopeless and wants to go home.

The Tool for Assessment of Suicide Risk: TASR

NAME: _____ Chart #: _____

INDIVIDUAL RISK PROFILE: ☆	YES	NO
Male		
Ages 15-35		
Age over 65		
Family history of suicide		
Chronic medical illness		
Psychiatric illness		
Poor social supports/social isolation		
Substance abuse		
Sexual/physical abuse		
SYMPTOM RISK PROFILE: ☆ ☆	**YES**	**NO**
Depressive symptoms		
Positive psychotic symptoms		
Hopelessness		
Worthlessness		
Anhedonia		
Anxiety/agitation		
Panic attacks		
Anger		
Impulsivity		
INTERVIEW RISK PROFILE: ☆ ☆ ☆	**YES**	**NO**
Recent substance use		
Suicidal ideation		
Suicidal intent		
Suicidal plan		
Access to lethal means		
Past suicide behaviour		
Current problems seem unsolvable to patient		
Suicidal/violent command hallucinations		

LEVEL OF SUICIDE RISK: High ☐   Moderate ☐   Low ☐

Assessment completed by: _____
(Name & position)
                                        DATE: _____

Case Seven

Mr J. is a 34-year-old male who telephones the clinic and says (with slurred speech) that he is suicidal. He states that he has a gun and has decided to kill himself after he kills his wife and 6-month-old child because 'they are possessed by the devil'. He wants the clinic doctor to come to the house and make sure that everyone is dead because that is the only way that he can think of to 'save their souls'.

The Tool for Assessment of Suicide Risk: TASR

NAME: _____ Chart #: _____

INDIVIDUAL RISK PROFILE: ☆	YES	NO
Male		
Ages 15-35		
Age over 65		
Family history of suicide		
Chronic medical illness		
Psychiatric illness		
Poor social supports/social isolation		
Substance abuse		
Sexual/physical abuse		

SYMPTOM RISK PROFILE: ☆ ☆	YES	NO
Depressive symptoms		
Positive psychotic symptoms		
Hopelessness		
Worthlessness		
Anhedonia		
Anxiety/agitation		
Panic attacks		
Anger		
Impulsivity		

INTERVIEW RISK PROFILE: ☆ ☆ ☆	YES	NO
Recent substance use		
Suicidal ideation		
Suicidal intent		
Suicidal plan		
Access to lethal means		
Past suicide behaviour		
Current problems seem unsolvable to patient		
Suicidal/violent command hallucinations		

LEVEL OF SUICIDE RISK: High ☐   Moderate ☐   Low ☐

Assessment completed by: _____
(Name & position)
                                    DATE: _____

© Dr. Stan Kutcher & Dr. Sonia Chehil, 2005

Case Eight

Mr R.J. is a 67-year-old bank executive and high-profile community leader. He is active in a number of health charities and is the financial controller at his church. He is well known to the hospital staff as he recently stepped down as chairman of the hospital board. This evening he presents to the emergency room with rapid onset of chest pain accompanied by respiratory distress, palpitations and thoughts that he will die. This episode came on suddenly as he and his wife were getting ready to go out to a cancer society fundraising dinner. It had largely resolved by the time he was assessed in the emergency room.

All investigations including EKG and cardiac enzymes are unremarkable. His wife, who had accompanied him to the hospital, has just left to 'go home and change clothes'. He asks to see you in private and confides that earlier that day he was informed by a physician in a confidential 'walk-in' clinic in a distant location in the city that he was HIV positive, the result of an eight-month secret relationship with one of the teenage girls (a known sex worker and intravenous drug abuser) whom he had been 'counselling' through a church-based programme for street youth. He has not told anyone about what has happened and a counsellor at the 'walk-in' clinic has asked him to come to an appointment tomorrow to discuss what he needs to do.

Mr R.J. has no personal or family history of mental illness and has never considered nor attempted suicide. He has had no significant medical illnesses and is taking no medications. However, since he received the news about his health status earlier today he has been having severe anxiety, numerous physical symptoms and is experiencing frequent suicidal thoughts that are intense but of short duration. He does not know what he should do. He is mortified at what this situation may do to his reputation and is convinced that he will be fired from his work. He feels guilty about his actions and does not know what he will tell his wife. He denies having a suicidal plan and does not want to keep his appointment at the clinic tomorrow, but instead thinks that he should 'go for a holiday to try and sort this out'.

The Tool for Assessment of Suicide Risk: TASR

NAME: _____   Chart #: _____

INDIVIDUAL RISK PROFILE: ☆	YES	NO
Male		
Ages 15-35		
Age over 65		
Family history of suicide		
Chronic medical illness		
Psychiatric illness		
Poor social supports/social isolation		
Substance abuse		
Sexual/physical abuse		
SYMPTOM RISK PROFILE: ☆ ☆	**YES**	**NO**
Depressive symptoms		
Positive psychotic symptoms		
Hopelessness		
Worthlessness		
Anhedonia		
Anxiety/agitation		
Panic attacks		
Anger		
Impulsivity		
INTERVIEW RISK PROFILE: ☆ ☆ ☆	**YES**	**NO**
Recent substance use		
Suicidal ideation		
Suicidal intent		
Suicidal plan		
Access to lethal means		
Past suicide behaviour		
Current problems seem unsolvable to patient		
Suicidal/violent command hallucinations		

LEVEL OF SUICIDE RISK: High ☐   Moderate ☐   Low ☐

Assessment completed by: _____
(Name & position)
                                    DATE: _____

© Dr. Stan Kutcher & Dr. Sonia Chehil, 2005

Appendices

The tools found in these appendices are to be used for clinical purposes by experienced clinicians or health/education professionals in patient/client assessment only. These tools are the copyright of the authors. Any other use of these tools requires written permission from the authors.

Suicide Risk Assessment Guide (SRAG)

SUICIDE RISK ASSESSMENT GUIDE: SRAG

NAME: _____ Chart #:_____ Age: _____ F / M

ADDRESS: _____

PHONE # Home: _____ Office: _____

CONTACT PERSON: _____ & PHONE: _____

☑ Check the boxes within each section that apply to the patient you have seen and rate the level of significance or severity of each of these factors to the patient from 1-3: **1= minimal 2= moderate 3=high**

		1	2	3
Current suicidal ideation	☐ Intensity	1	2	3
	☐ Frequency	1	2	3
	☐ Persistence	1	2	3
Current suicide intent & plan	☐ Expectation & commitment to die	1	2	3
	☐ Lethality of method	1	2	3
	☐ Availability of means	1	2	3
	☐ Patient's belief in lethality of method	1	2	3
	☐ Chance of rescue	1	2	3
	☐ Steps taken to enact plan	1	2	3
	☐ Preparedness for death	1	2	3

High lethality

Low frequency — High frequency

Low lethality

⬇

Past self-harm behaviours

Suicide Motivation: *Why & Why Not?*

	Number	Lethality		
☐ Past suicide attempts		1	2	3
☐ Past self-harm behaviours		1	2	3

Symptom risk factors

Current high risk symptoms

Ø psychiatric disorder — + psychiatric disorder

Ø current high risk symptoms

		1	2	3
☐ Hopelessness		1	2	3
☐ Significant anxiety/panic attacks		1	2	3
☐ Command hallucinations		1	2	3
☐ Impulsivity		1	2	3
☐ Aggression		1	2	3
☐ Dysphoria		1	2	3
☐ Anhedonia		1	2	3
☐ Shame or humiliation		1	2	3
☐ Decreased self-esteem		1	2	3
☐ Agitation		1	2	3
☐ Akathisia		1	2	3
☐ Anger		1	2	3
☐ Severe insomnia		1	2	3

1

Suicide risk factors (SRFs) for patients with ANY psychiatric disorder	☐ Social isolation	1	2	3
	☐ Loss of family role/status	1	2	3
	☐ Interpersonal losses	1	2	3
	☐ Vocational/occupational loss	1	2	3
	☐ Loss of previous skills/competencies	1	2	3
	☐ Awareness of deficits with recovery	1	2	3
	☐ Substance or alcohol abuse/dependence	1	2	3
	☐ ↓ Problem solving capacity (cognitive impairment)	1	2	3
	☐ Depressive symptoms	1	2	3
	☐ Hopelessness	1	2	3

☹ Depression symptom checklist	☐ Low mood	1	2	3
	☐ ↓ Interest in activities/↓ ability to feel pleasure	1	2	3
	☐ Significant change in weight	1	2	3
	☐ Sleep difficulties	1	2	3
	☐ Restless or slowed down	1	2	3
	☐ Fatigue/↓ energy	1	2	3
	☐ Feelings of worthlessness/guilt	1	2	3
	☐ Poor concentration or difficulty making decisions	1	2	3

Additional SRFs for patients with depression	☐ Significant anxiety/panic attacks	1	2	3
	☐ Anhedonia	1	2	3
	☐ Psychosis	1	2	3
	☐ Return of energy early in recovery	1	2	3
	☐ Sudden clinical improvement	1	2	3

☹ Anxiety symptom checklist	☐ Excessive worry	1	2	3
	☐ Has difficulty controlling worry			
	☐ Restlessness	1	2	3
	☐ Fatigue	1	2	3
	☐ Poor concentration	1	2	3
	☐ Irritability	1	2	3
	☐ Muscle tension	1	2	3
	☐ Poor sleep (falling asleep/↑awakening at night)	1	2	3
	☐ Panic attacks	1	2	3

Additional SRFs for patients with anxiety	☐ Panic attacks	1	2	3

Additional SRFs for patients with schizophrenia	☐ Recent hospital discharge	1	2	3
	☐ Recovery following acute psychotic episode	1	2	3
	☐ Suicidal/violent command hallucinations	1	2	3
	☐ Akathisia	1	2	3
	☐ Agitation	1	2	3

Current substance use: ☐ Alcohol ☐ Cannabis ☐ Other: _____

Substance use d/o symptom checklist:	☐ ↑ Problematic use	1	2	3
	☐ Use despite significant/recurrent consequences	1	2	3
	☐ Tolerance	1	2	3
	☐ Withdrawal	1	2	3
	☐ Past history abuse or dependence	1	2	3

Additional SRFs for patients with any SUD	☐ Recent, threatened or impending interpersonal loss	1	2	3
	☐ Presence of other psychiatric disorder	1	2	3
	☐ Presence of a depressive episode	1	2	3

Additional SRFs for patients with alcohol use d/o	☐ Continued or heavier drinking	1	2	3
	☐ Serious medical illness	1	2	3
	☐ Personality disturbance/psychiatric disorder	1	2	3
	☐ Other substance use	1	2	3

Risk factors for patients with medical disorders	☐ Chronic disease	1	2	3
	☐ Neurological disorder	1	2	3
	☐ Pain	1	2	3
	☐ Functional impairment	1	2	3
	☐ Cognitive impairment	1	2	3
	☐ Loss of sight or hearing	1	2	3
	☐ Disfigurement	1	2	3
	☐ Increased dependency on others	1	2	3
	☐ Presence of psychiatric disorder or symptoms	1	2	3

Family risk factors

Strong history mental d/o or suicide

Supportive ← → Abusive

Ø history mental d/o or suicide

	☐ Suicide or suicide attempts in family	1	2	3
	☐ Suicide or suicide attempts in 1st degree relative	1	2	3
	☐ Psychiatric disorder in family	1	2	3
	☐ Psychiatric disorder in 1st degree relative	1	2	3
	☐ Substance use disorder in family	1	2	3
	☐ Domestic violence/abuse	1	2	3
	☐ ↑ Family conflict	1	2	3

Psychosocial risk factors

No supports

Ø sign. stressor ← → ++ stressors

++ supports

	☐ Actual/perceived interpersonal loss/bereavement	1	2	3
	☐ Financial difficulties	1	2	3
	☐ Changes in socio-economic status	1	2	3
	☐ Family problems	1	2	3
	☐ Marital/relationship problems	1	2	3
	☐ Interpersonal/peer group problem	1	2	3
	☐ Domestic violence	1	2	3
	☐ Past or current abuse or neglect	1	2	3
	☐ Housing problems	1	2	3
	☐ Work/school problems	1	2	3
	☐ Legal difficulties	1	2	3
	☐ Perceived humiliation	1	2	3

3

Personality risk factors				
	☐ History of poor coping skills	1	2	3
Rigid/impulsive poor coping	☐ History of poor problem solving	1	2	3
	☐ Impulsivity	1	2	3
Hopeful ⟷ Hopeless	☐ Poor insight	1	2	3
	☐ Poor affective control	1	2	3
	☐ Rigid thinking	1	2	3
Flexible/adaptive good coping	☐ Dependency	1	2	3
	☐ Manipulative	1	2	3

SUICIDE RISK ASSESSMENT SUMMARY:

SUICIDE RISK PROFILE	SYMPTOM RISK PROFILE	INTERVIEW RISK PROFILE
☐ Male	☐ Depressive symptoms	☐ Recent substance use
☐ Ages 15-35	☐ Positive psychotic symptoms	☐ Suicidal ideation
☐ Age over 65	☐ Hopelessness	☐ Suicidal intent
☐ Family history of suicide	☐ Worthlessness	☐ Suicidal plan
☐ Chronic medical illness	☐ Anhedonia	☐ Access to lethal means
☐ Psychiatric illness	☐ Anxiety/agitation	☐ Past suicide behaviour
☐ Poor social supports/isolation	☐ Panic attacks	☐ Current problems seem
☐ Substance abuse	☐ Anger	unsolvable to patient
☐ Sexual/physical abuse	☐ Impulsivity	☐ Command hallucinations

Risk profile rating			**Symptom profile rating**			**Interview profile rating**		
Low	Moderate	High	Low	Moderate	High	Low	Moderate	High
☐	☐	☐	☐	☐	☐	☐	☐	☐

IMPRESSION & PLAN: _____

_____

_____

_____

_____

_____

_____

_____

_____

_____

_____

_____

Clinician name: _____   **Date:** _____

4

Tool for Assessment of Suicide Risk (TASR)

The Tool for Assessment of Suicide Risk: TASR

NAME: _____ Chart #: _____

INDIVIDUAL RISK PROFILE: ☆	YES	NO
Male		
Ages 15-35		
Age over 65		
Family history of suicide		
Chronic medical illness		
Psychiatric illness		
Poor social supports/social isolation		
Substance abuse		
Sexual/physical abuse		
SYMPTOM RISK PROFILE: ☆ ☆	**YES**	**NO**
Depressive symptoms		
Positive psychotic symptoms		
Hopelessness		
Worthlessness		
Anhedonia		
Anxiety/agitation		
Panic attacks		
Anger		
Impulsivity		
INTERVIEW RISK PROFILE: ☆ ☆ ☆	**YES**	**NO**
Recent substance use		
Suicidal ideation		
Suicidal intent		
Suicidal plan		
Access to lethal means		
Past suicide behaviour		
Current problems seem unsolvable to patient		
Suicidal/violent command hallucinations		

LEVEL OF SUICIDE RISK: High ☐   Moderate ☐   Low ☐

Assessment completed by: _____
(Name & position)
                                   DATE: _____

© Dr. Stan Kutcher & Dr. Sonia Chehil, 2005

6-item Kutcher Adolescent Depression Scale (KADS)

6-ITEM Kutcher Adolescent Depression Scale: KADS-6

NAME: _____ CHART NUMBER: _____

DATE: _____ ASSESSMENT COMPLETED BY: _____

OVER THE LAST WEEK, HOW HAVE YOU BEEN "ON AVERAGE" OR "USUALLY" REGARDING THE FOLLOWING ITEMS:

1. **Low mood, sadness, feeling blah or down, depressed, just can't be bothered.**

   ☐ 0 - Hardly ever   ☐ 1 - Much of the time   ☐ 2 - Most of the time   ☐ 3 - All of the time

2. **Feelings of worthlessness, hopelessness, letting people down, not being a good person.**

   ☐ 0 - Hardly ever   ☐ 1 - Much of the time   ☐ 2 - Most of the time   ☐ 3 - All of the time

3. **Feeling tired, feeling fatigued, low in energy, hard to get motivated, have to push to get things done, want to rest or lie down a lot.**

   ☐ 0 - Hardly ever   ☐ 1 - Much of the time   ☐ 2 - Most of the time   ☐ 3 - All of the time

4. **Feeling that life is not very much fun, not feeling good when usually (before getting sick) would feel good, not getting as much pleasure from fun things as usual (before getting sick).**

   ☐ 0 - Hardly ever   ☐ 1 - Much of the time   ☐ 2 - Most of the time   ☐ 3 - All of the time

5. **Feeling worried, nervous, panicky, tense, keyed up, anxious.**

   ☐ 0 - Hardly ever   ☐ 1 - Much of the time   ☐ 2 - Most of the time   ☐ 3 - All of the time

6. **Thoughts, plans or actions about suicide or self-harm.**

   ☐ 0 - Hardly ever   ☐ 1 - Much of the time   ☐ 2 - Most of the time   ☐ 3 - All of the time

TOTAL SCORE: _____

1

6-ITEM Kutcher Adolescent Depression Scale: KADS-6

OVERVIEW

The Kutcher Adolescent Depression Scale (KADS) is a **self-report** scale specifically designed to diagnosis and assess the severity of adolescent depression, and versions include a 16-item, an 11 item and an abbreviated 6-item scale.

SCORING INSTRUCTIONS

TOTAL SCORE	SCORE INTERPRETATION
0–5	Probably not depressed
6 and ABOVE	Possible depression; more thorough assessment needed

REFERENCE

LeBlanc JC, Almudevar A, Brooks SJ, Kutcher S: Screening for Adolescent Depression: Comparison of the Kutcher Adolescent Depression Scale with the Beck Depression Inventory, Journal of Child and Adolescent Psychopharmacology, 2002 Summer; 12(2):113-26.

Self-report instruments commonly used to assess depression in adolescents have limited or unknown reliability and validity in this age group. We describe a new self-report scale, the Kutcher Adolescent Depression Scale (KADS), designed specifically to diagnose and assess the severity of adolescent depression. This report compares the diagnostic validity of the full 16-item instrument, brief versions of it, and the Beck Depression Inventory (BDI) against the criteria for major depressive episode (MDE) from the Mini International Neuropsychiatric Interview (MINI). Some 309 of 1,712 grade 7 to grade 12 students who completed the BDI had scores that exceeded 15. All were invited for further assessment, of whom 161 agreed to assessment by the KADS, the BDI again, and a MINI diagnostic interview for MDE. Receiver operating characteristic (ROC) curve analysis was used to determine which KADS items best identified subjects experiencing an MDE. *Further ROC curve analyses established that the overall diagnostic ability of a six-item subscale of the KADS was at least as good as that of the BDI and was better than that of the full-length KADS. Used with a cut-off score of 6, the six-item KADS achieved sensitivity and specificity rates of 92% and 71%, respectively—a combination not achieved by other self-report instruments. The six-item KADS may prove to be an efficient and effective means of ruling out MDE in adolescents.*

2

11-ITEM Kutcher Adolescent Depression Scale: KADS-11

NAME: _____ CHART NUMBER: _____

DATE: _____ ASSESSMENT COMPLETED BY: _____

OVER THE LAST WEEK, HOW HAVE YOU BEEN "ON AVERAGE" OR "USUALLY" REGARDING THE FOLLOWING ITEMS:

1. **Low mood, sadness, feeling blah or down, depressed, just can't be bothered.**

   ☐   ☐   ☐   ☐
   0 - Hardly ever   1 - Much of the time 2 - Most of the time 3 - All of the time

2. **Irritable, losing your temper easily, feeling pissed off, losing it.**

   ☐   ☐   ☐   ☐
   0 - Hardly ever   1 - Much of the time 2 - Most of the time 3 - All of the time

3. **Sleep Difficulties - different from your usual (over the years before you got sick): trouble falling asleep, lying awake in bed.**

   ☐   ☐   ☐   ☐
   0 - Hardly ever   1 - Much of the time 2 - Most of the time 3 - All of the time

4. **Feeling Decreased Interest In: hanging out with friends; being with your best friend; being with your partner / boyfriend / girlfriend; going out of the house; doing school work or work; doing hobbies or sports or recreation.**

   ☐   ☐   ☐   ☐
   0 - Hardly ever   1 - Much of the time 2 - Most of the time 3 - All of the time

5. **Feelings of worthlessness, hopelessness, letting people down, not being a good person.**

   ☐   ☐   ☐   ☐
   0 - Hardly ever   1 - Much of the time 2 - Most of the time 3 - All of the time

1

Dr. Stan Kutcher, 2006

6. **Feeling tired, feeling fatigued, low in energy, hard to get motivated, have to push to get things done, want to rest or lie down a lot.**

☐ 0 - Hardly ever   ☐ 1 - Much of the time   ☐ 2 - Most of the time   ☐ 3 - All of the time

7. **Trouble concentrating, can't keep your mind on schoolwork or work, daydreaming when you should be working, hard to focus when reading, getting "bored" with work or school.**

☐ 0 - Hardly ever   ☐ 1 - Much of the time   ☐ 2 - Most of the time   ☐ 3 - All of the time

8. **Feeling that life is not very much fun, not feeling good when usually (before getting sick) would feel good, not getting as much pleasure from fun things as usual (before getting sick).**

☐ 0 - Hardly ever   ☐ 1 - Much of the time   ☐ 2 - Most of the time   ☐ 3 - All of the time

9. **Feeling worried, nervous, panicky, tense, keyed up, anxious.**

☐ 0 - Hardly ever   ☐ 1 - Much of the time   ☐ 2 - Most of the time   ☐ 3 - All of the time

10. **Physical feelings of worry like: headaches, butterflies, nausea, tingling, restlessness, diarrhoea, shakes or tremors.**

☐ 0 - Hardly ever   ☐ 1 - Much of the time   ☐ 2 - Most of the time   ☐ 3 - All of the time

11. **Thoughts, plans or actions about suicide or self-harm.**

☐ 0 - No thoughts or plans or actions   ☐ 1 - Occasional thoughts, no plans or actions   ☐ 2 - Frequent thoughts, no plans or actions   ☐ 3 - Plans and/or actions that have hurt

TOTAL SCORE: ☐

2

Dr. Stan Kutcher, 2006

11-ITEM Kutcher Adolescent Depression Scale: KADS-11

OVERVIEW

The Kutcher Adolescent Depression Scale (KADS) is a **self-report** scale specifically designed to diagnosis and assess the severity of adolescent depression, and versions include a 16-item, a 11-item and an abbreviated 6-item scale.

SCORING INTERPRETATION

There are no validated diagnostic categories associated with particular ranges of scores. All scores should be assessed relative to an individual patient's baseline score (higher scores indicating worsening depression, lower scores suggesting possible improvement).

REFERENCE

LeBlanc JC, Almudevar A, Brooks SJ, Kutcher S: Screening for Adolescent Depression: Comparison of the Kutcher Adolescent Depression Scale with the Beck Depression Inventory, Journal of Child and Adolescent Psychopharmacology, 2002 Summer; 12(2):113-26.

Self-report instruments commonly used to assess depression in adolescents have limited or unknown reliability and validity in this age group. We describe a new self-report scale, the Kutcher Adolescent Depression Scale (KADS), designed specifically to diagnose and assess the severity of adolescent depression. This report compares the diagnostic validity of the full 16-item instrument, brief versions of it, and the Beck Depression Inventory (BDI) against the criteria for major depressive episode (MDE) from the Mini International Neuropsychiatric Interview (MINI). Some 309 of 1,712 grade 7 to grade 12 students who completed the BDI had scores that exceeded 15. All were invited for further assessment, of whom 161 agreed to assessment by the KADS, the BDI again, and a MINI diagnostic interview for MDE. Receiver operating characteristic (ROC) curve analysis was used to determine which KADS items best identified subjectsexperiencing an MDE. *Further ROC curve analyses established that the overall diagnostic ability of a six-item subscale of the KADS was at least as good as that of the BDI and was better than that of the full-length KADS. Used with a cut-off score of 6, the six-item KADS achieved sensitivity and specificity rates of 92% and 71%, respectively—a combination not achieved by other self-report instruments. The six-item KADS may prove to be an efficient and effective means of ruling out MDE in adolescents.*

3

Dr. Stan Kutcher, 2006

Appendix 4

Chehil and Kutcher Clinical Assessment of Adolescent Depression (CAAD)

NAME: _____ Chart # _____ Date: _____

INFORMANT: _____ Tele: _____

Chehil & Kutcher CLINICAL ASSESSMENT OF ADOLESCENT DEPRESSION (CAAD)

Record the frequency of occurrence OVER THE PAST ONE WEEK for each symptom below then rate the symptom on a 4 point scale (0-3) in the *symptom* column. Document relevant clinical information in the *Clinician Review* column (i.e. course, aggravating/mitigating factors, impact on home/school/recreational functioning, etc.) and rate the symptom from 0-3 based on the composite information obtained.

Symptom rating:
0 = Does not bother the adolescent
1 = Mild distress and no significant impairment in home, school, or social function
2 = Moderate distress and some impairment in home, school, or social function
3 = Severe distress and significant impairment in home, school, or social function

SYMPTOM: Low mood, sadness, blah, down, depressed, just can't be bothered.

Over the past week I have experienced this:	Patient symptom rating (0-3)	Informant symptom rating (0-3)	Clinician composite symptom rating (0-3)
☐ Hardly ever ☐ Much of the time ☐ Most of the time ☐ All of the time			

Notes:

SYMPTOM: Irritable, losing temper easily, feeling pissed off, losing it.

Over the past week I have experienced this:	Patient symptom rating (0-3)	Informant symptom rating (0-3)	Clinician composite symptom rating (0-3)
☐ Hardly ever ☐ Much of the time ☐ Most of the time ☐ All of the time			

Notes:

1

© Dr Sonia Chehil & Dr Stan Kutcher

SYMPTOM: Sleep difficulties - different from usual (over the years before getting sick): trouble falling asleep, lying awake in bed.

Over the past week I have experienced this:	Patient symptom rating (0-3)	Informant symptom rating (0-3)	Clinician composite symptom rating (0-3)
☐ Hardly ever ☐ Much of the time ☐ Most of the time ☐ All of the time			

Notes:

SYMPTOM: Decreased interest in: being with friends/best friend/partner/boy or girl friend; going out; school work; work; hobbies; sports; recreation.

Over the past week I have experienced this:	Patient symptom rating (0-3)	Informant symptom rating (0-3)	Clinician composite symptom rating (0-3)
☐ Hardly ever ☐ Much of the time ☐ Most of the time ☐ All of the time			

Notes:

SYMPTOM: Sense of worthlessness, hopelessness, letting people down, not being a good person.

Over the past week I have experienced this:	Patient symptom rating (0-3)	Informant symptom rating (0-3)	Clinician composite symptom rating (0-3)
☐ Hardly ever ☐ Much of the time ☐ Most of the time ☐ All of the time			

Notes:

2

SYMPTOM: Tired, fatigued, low in energy, hard to get motivated, have to push to get things done, want to rest or lie down a lot.

Over the past week I have experienced this:	Patient symptom rating (0-3)	Informant symptom rating (0-3)	Clinician composite symptom rating (0-3)
☐ Hardly ever ☐ Much of the time ☐ Most of the time ☐ All of the time			

Notes:

SYMPTOM: Trouble concentrating, can't keep mind on school/work, daydreaming, hard to focus when reading, getting 'bored' with work or school.

Over the past week I have experienced this:	Patient symptom rating (0-3)	Informant symptom rating (0-3)	Clinician composite symptom rating (0-3)
☐ Hardly ever ☐ Much of the time ☐ Most of the time ☐ All of the time			

Notes:

SYMPTOM: Life is not very much fun, not able to enjoy things once enjoyed, not getting as much pleasure from fun things as before getting sick.

Over the past week I have experienced this:	Patient symptom rating (0-3)	Informant symptom rating (0-3)	Clinician composite symptom rating (0-3)
☐ Hardly ever ☐ Much of the time ☐ Most of the time ☐ All of the time			

Notes:

3

© Dr Sonia Chehil & Dr Stan Kutcher

SYMPTOM: Worried, nervous, panicky, tense, keyed up, anxious.			
Over the past week I have experienced this: ☐ Hardly ever ☐ Much of the time ☐ Most of the time ☐ All of the time	**Patient symptom rating (0-3)**	**Informant symptom rating (0-3)**	**Clinician composite symptom rating (0-3)**

Notes:

SYMPTOM: Physical expression of worry: headaches, butterflies, knots in the stomach, nausea, tingling, restlessness, diarrhoea, shakiness.			
Over the past week I have experienced this: ☐ Hardly ever ☐ Much of the time ☐ Most of the time ☐ All of the time	**Patient symptom rating (0-3)**	**Informant symptom rating (0-3)**	**Clinician composite symptom rating (0-3)**

Notes:

SYMPTOM: Thoughts, plans or actions about suicide or self-harm.		
Over the past week I have experienced this: ☐ No thoughts or plans or actions ☐ Occasional thoughts, no plans or actions ☐ Frequent thoughts, no plans or actions ☐ Plans and/or actions that have hurt	**Patient symptom rating (0-3)**	**Clinician composite symptom rating (0-3)**

☑ RISK FACTOR	YES	NO
☐ Suicidal ideation		
☐ Suicidal intent		
☐ Suicidal plan		
☐ Access to lethal means		
☐ Past suicide behaviour		
☐ Problems seem unsolvable		
☐ Hopelessness/worthlessness		
☐ Anger/impulsivity		

Notes:

4

Substance use: NO ☐   YES ☐   list: _____

Current substance use:

☐ None in the last 1 month
☐ 1 substance once weekly or less
☐ 1 substance 2-3x/week or 2 substances 1-2x/week
☐ 1 substance 4x/week or 2 substances 2-3x/week or polysubstance use (>3 substances)

Patient symptom rating (0-3)	Informant symptom rating (0-3)	Clinician composite symptom rating (0-3)
☐	☐	☐

Notes:

CLINICAL SUMMARY	PATIENT RATING				INFORMANT RATING				CLINICIAN RATING			
SYMPTOMS	0	1	2	3	0	1	2	3	0	1	2	3
SIDE EFFECTS	0	1	2	3	0	1	2	3	0	1	2	3
SCHOOL/WORK FUNCTION	0	1	2	3	0	1	2	3	0	1	2	3
FAMILY FUNCTION	0	1	2	3	0	1	2	3	0	1	2	3
PEER FUNCTION	0	1	2	3	0	1	2	3	0	1	2	3
RECREATION FUNCTION	0	1	2	3	0	1	2	3	0	1	2	3
SAFETY	0	1	2	3	0	1	2	3	0	1	2	3
OVERALL SUMMARY RATING:	0	1	2	3	0	1	2	3	0	1	2	3

PATIENT FOLLOW-UP ASSESSMENT															
CLINICAL CHANGE RATING	Rate change since last assessment based on patient, informant and clinician impression (-2 to +2) -2: much worse -1: little worse 0: no change +1: little better +2: much better														
DOMAIN	PATIENT RATING					INFORMANT RATING					CLINICIAN RATING				
SYMPTOMS	-2	-1	0	+1	+2	-2	-1	0	+1	+2	-2	-1	0	+1	+2
SIDE EFFECTS	-2	-1	0	+1	+2	-2	-1	0	+1	+2	-2	-1	0	+1	+2
SCHOOL/WORK FUNCTION	-2	-1	0	+1	+2	-2	-1	0	+1	+2	-2	-1	0	+1	+2
FAMILY FUNCTION	-2	-1	0	+1	+2	-2	-1	0	+1	+2	-2	-1	0	+1	+2
PEER FUNCTION	-2	-1	0	+1	+2	-2	-1	0	+1	+2	-2	-1	0	+1	+2
RECREATION FUNCTION	-2	-1	0	+1	+2	-2	-1	0	+1	+2	-2	-1	0	+1	+2
SAFETY	-2	-1	0	+1	+2	-2	-1	0	+1	+2	-2	-1	0	+1	+2
SUMMARY (since last assessment)	-2	-1	0	+1	+2	-2	-1	0	+1	+2	-2	-1	0	+1	+2
OVERALL IMPROVEMENT Since initiation of intervention or mental health contact	Patient overall rating					Informant overall rating					Clinician overall rating				
	-2	-1	0	+1	+2	-2	-1	0	+1	+2	-2	-1	0	+1	+2

5

Medical dx & concerns: _____
_____
_____

Current medications: include all prescription, herbal, vitamin, over-the-counter medicines.

Notes:_____
_____
_____
_____
_____
_____
_____
_____
_____
_____
_____
_____
_____
_____
_____
_____
_____
_____
_____
_____
_____
_____
_____

IMPRESSION & PLAN: _____
_____
_____
_____
_____
_____
_____

REFERRAL/DISPOSITION: _____

F/U CLINICIAN: _____ DATE/TIME: _____

ASSESSMENT COMPLETED BY: _____ **Sign:** _____

6

Index

abuse, physical
  see also alcohol abuse; substance use
  risk factor 9, 27, 28
adolescence 7
  see also youth
  CAAD 79, 124–9
age, risk factor 7–8, 12
AIDS *see* HIV/AIDS
alcohol abuse
  see also substance use
  assessment 58
  clinical vignette 100
  risk factor 12, 21–2
anxiety attacks, clinical vignettes 98, 110
anxiety disorders
  assessment 57
  risk factor 20
assessment of suicidality, risk assessment 38, 40–4
assessment, risk *see* risk assessment
avoid, approaches to 41–2
awareness lack 4

barriers
  detection 2–5
  prevention 2–5
basic principles, intervention 88–92
behavioural responses 81–5
breast cancer, clinical vignette 106

CAAD *see* Clinical Assessment of Adolescent Depression
cancer, clinical vignette 106

cases, risk assessment 96–111
Chehil and Kutcher Clinical Assessment of Adolescent Depression (CAAD) *see* Clinical Assessment of Adolescent Depression
chronically suicidal patients 80–5
Clinical Assessment of Adolescent Depression (CAAD) 124–9
  youth 79
clinical vignettes 96–111
cognitive responses 81–5
collateral history, youth 76
collateral information 43–4
communication 2, 3
  lack 4
  rapport 40–1
confidentiality, youth 76
context, suicide vi–vii
contract, suicide prevention 90
correlation, mental disorders/suicide 2
counselling, post-suicide interventions 94
country comparisons 1
cultural beliefs 27–8
current suicidality, risk factor 12–15

deaths, homicide/suicide 1
demographics, risk factors 7–12
depression
  assessment 56, 77, 79
  clinical vignettes 96, 100, 106
  KADS 77, 119–23
  risk factor 15–18
  youth 71–3, 77, 79

detection, barriers 2–5
difficult patients 80–5

education, post-suicide interventions 94–5
elderly people 7–8
emotional responses 81–5
empathic statements 41
employment status
   clinical vignettes 98, 100
   risk factor 26–7
evaluation of risk factors, risk assessment
      39, 52–65
evaluation of suicide risk, problems 80–5

family history
   assessment 60–1
   risk factor 24–5
   youth 76
frequency, past/current suicidality 48
frequent attempters 80–5

gender, risk factor 8–12
gentle inquiry 41
gun, clinical vignette 108

hallucinations, risk factor 19–20
help, failure to seek 4
hidden psychiatric disorders 83–4
histories
   collateral 76
   family 24–5, 60–1, 76
   individual 23–9, 76
   medical 23–4
   psychosocial 25–8, 61–3
HIV/AIDS
   clinical vignette 110
   risk factor 24
homicide deaths, cf. suicide deaths 1
hopelessness 18, 22, 35, 36, 42, 53–4

ideation, suicidal
   assessment 44
   risk factor 13, 15
incidence, suicide 1–2
individual histories, risk factors 23–9, 76
individual risk profile, TASR 68

individual strategies 86–7
intent, suicidal
   assessment 45–7, 61
   risk factor 13, 15
intervention programmes, youth 86–7
interventions 88–92
   basic principles 88–92
   post-suicide 93–5
   risk assessment 40
   safety/security 88–9
   support 89–90
   targeted 91–2
interview profile, TASR 69

KADS see Kutcher Adolescent Depression
      Scale
knowledge lack 4
Kutcher Adolescent Depression Scale
      (KADS) 119–23
   youth 77

learning, post-suicide interventions 94
low-lethality attempters 80–5

management principles, intervention
      88–92
marital status, risk factor 26
medical disorders, assessment 58
medical history, risk factor 23–4
mental disorders, suicide correlation 2
mood disorders, risk factor 17–18
motivations, suicide, assessment 46
myths 3

need, risk assessment 36
neurobiology 29
'no harm' contract 90

objectives, this book's viii
objectivity 83–5
overall rating, assessment 70
overwhelming feelings 84

past/current suicidality
   assessment 48–52
   frequency 48

lethality 49
nature/severity 49–51
risk factor 12–15
types 48
personality disorders, risk factor 22
personality strengths/weaknesses
assessment 63–4
risk factor 29–30
plans, suicidal
assessment 45–6
risk factor 14–15
population strategies 86–7
post-suicide interventions 93–5
postpartum depression 10–11
postpartum psychosis (PPP) 11
predicting suicide 5
prevalence, suicide 1–2
prevention
barriers 2–5
strategies 86–7
principles, intervention 88–92
problems, evaluation of suicide risk 80–5
protective factors 5–6
psychiatric disorders
hidden 83–4
risk factor 2, 15–22
summary 22
psychiatric symptoms, risk factor 15–17
psychosocial history
assessment 61–3
risk factor 25–8
psychotic disorders, risk factor 19–20

rapport 40–1
rarity, suicide 4–5
rates, suicide 1–2, 7
'reasons for living', protective factor 28
reasons, suicide vi–vii
religious beliefs 2, 6, 27–8
risk assessment 34–65
assessment of suicidality 38, 40–4
clinical vignettes 96–111
evaluation of risk factors 39, 52–65
intervention 40
need 36
practice cases 96–111

prevented 89
SRAG 34–65, 114–17
steps summary 38–40
summary 65
TASR 66–70, 96–111, 118
timing 36–7
what's going on? 39
youth, summary 78
risk factors 5–33
demographics 7–12
histories, individual 23–9, 76
past/current suicidality 12–15
personality strengths/weaknesses 29–30
psychiatric disorders 2, 15–22
summary 31–3

safety/security, intervention 88–9
schizophrenia
assessment 57
risk factor 19–20
self-harm behaviours 83–5
clinical vignettes 102, 104
SRAG 51–2
sexual orientation, risk factor 25
social stigma 2–3
specific serotonin reuptake inhibitors
(SSRIs), youth 77
SRAG see Suicide Risk Assessment Guide
SSRIs see specific serotonin reuptake
inhibitors
stigma 2–3
strategies, prevention 86–7
substance use
see also alcohol abuse
assessment 57–8
clinical vignette 104
risk factor 21–2
suicide prevention contract 90
Suicide Risk Assessment Guide (SRAG)
34–65, 114–17
support
intervention 89–90
post-suicide interventions 93
symptom profile, TASR 68–9

targeted interventions 91–2

TASR *see* Tool for Assessment of Suicide
    Risk
teenage *see* adolescence; youth
timing, risk assessment 36–7
Tool for Assessment of Suicide Risk
        (TASR) 66–70, 118
    clinical vignettes 96–111

unemployment
    clinical vignettes 98, 100
    risk factor 26–7

vignettes, clinical 96–111

warning signs, youth 73–5
weapon, clinical vignette 108

what's going on?, risk assessment 39

youth 71–9
    see also adolescence
    assessment summary 78
    CAAD 79, 124–9
    collateral history 76
    confidentiality 76
    depression 71–3, 77, 79
    disturbance cf. distress 73
    family history 76
    intervention programmes 86–7
    KADS 77
    prevention strategies 86–7
    SSRIs 77
    warning signs 73–5